HEALT

THE 50 MIRACLE CURES OF CURCUMIN

FAST SOLUTIONS FOR DIABETES, HIGH BLOOD PRESSURE, CHOLESTEROL, HEART, SLIMMING, KIDNEY, LIVER, JOINTS, ULCER, COLO, HIV/AIDS ALZHEIMER'S, MS, HEPATITIS, ACNE, UTI, HERPES GALLSTONES, ASHTMA, PSORIASIS, ……..

BY

Professor Awad Mansour

Professor of Chemical & Pharmaceutical Engineering
Formerly with
University of Akron
OH, U.S.A.

First Edition
2010

HEALTH TECH BOOK SERIES
9923 S. Ridgeland Ave. STE 209
Chicago Ridge, IL. 60415

Copyright @ 2010 by Professor Awad Mansour

All rights reserved, including the rights of reproduction in whole or in part in any form.

HEALTH TECH BOOK SERIES

Published and Printed in the United States by:
Health Tech Book Series

Mansour, Awad
THE 50 MIRACLE CURES OF CURCUMIN

First Edition

ISBN 1452879842
EAN: 9781452879840

HEALTH DISCLAIMER

THE 50 MIRACLE CURES OF CURCUMIN: IS DESIGNED FOR INFORMATIVE PURPOSES ONLY AND ANY READER IS EXPECTED TO CONSULT HIS FAMILY DOCTOR BEFORE TAKING ANY CHEMICAL OR NATURAL PRODUCTS AND THE AUTHOR IS NOT RESPONSIBLE FOR THE USE OR MISUSE OF THE INFORMATION CONTAINED WITHIN.

Table of Content

- ITRODUCTION 5
- CURCUMIN AND ACNE 7
- CURCUMIN AND ANEMIA 9
- CURCUMIN AND ARTHRITIS 13
- CURCUMIN AND BLADDER INFECTION 17
- CURCUMIN AND BODY ODOR & BAD BREATH 21
- CURCUMIN AND CANCER 24
- CURCUMIN AND CELLULITE 31
- CURCUMIN AND CHOLESTEROL 35
- CURCUMIN AND CONSTIPATION 39
- CURCUMIN AND DENGUE FEVER 43
- CURCUMIN AND DIABETES 45
- CURCUMIN AND DIGESTION 49
- CURCUMIN AND DYSENTRY 51
- CURCUMIN AND EYE CATARACT 53
- CURCUMIN AND FEVER 55
- CURCUMIN AND GOUT 57
- CURCUMIN AND HAIR LOSS 61
- CURCUMIN AND HEART HEALTH 63
- CURCUMIN AND HEMORROHIDS 67
- CURCUMIN AND HYPERTENSION 71
- CURCUMIN AND INSOMNIA 75
- CURCUMIN AND IRRITABLE COLON 77
- CURCUMIN AND JAUNDICE 79
- CURCUMIN AND KIDNEY HEALTH 81
- CURCUMIN AND LIVER CIRRHOSIS 83

CURCUMIN AND LOST APPETITE	89
CURCUMIN AND MEMORY	91
CURCUMIN AND MENSTRUAL FLOW PROBLEMS	93
CURCUMIN AND MOUTH ULCER	95
CURCUMIN AND MULTIPLE SCLEROSIS	99
CURCUMIN AND NOSE BLEED	103
CURCUMIN AND ODEMA (SWELLING)	105
CURCUMIN AND PIMPLES, BLACKHEADS AND DRY SKIN	109
CURCUMIN AND PROSTATE HEALTH	111
CURCUMIN AND PROSTATITIS	115
CURCUMIN AND PSORIASIS	117
CURCUMIN AND SEX	121
CURCUMIN AND SMALLPOX	125
CURCUMIN AND SORE THROAT	127
CURCUMIN AND TRIGLYCERIDES	129
CURCUMIN AND ULCER	133
CURCUMIN AND URINARY TRACT INFECTION (UTI)	135
CURCUMIN AND WEIGHT LOSS	137
CURCUMIN AS AN EFFICIENT HEAVY METALS DETOX	139
CURCUMIN CABBAGE MIRACLE SLIMMING SOUP	141
CURCUMIN LICE AND DANDRUFF	143
CURCUMIN, NAUSEA AND VOMITING	145
CURCUMIN IN PERFUMES, FLAVORS & NATURAL DYE INDUSTRY	147
CURCUMIN & SMART ICE CREAM Secret Formula	149
Phytochemical Compounds Inside Turmeric & Their Effects on Health	151
About the Author	

INTRODUCTION
Why I Wrote This Book?

The major reason behind writing this book about CURCUMIN is the continuous success stories I received from my patients about the miracle results of using coriander for numerous health conditions; one of these unique stories is the one found by my favorite patient Dr. Suher Yazbak from Palestine who suffered from **rheumatic psoriasis** severe conditions for years!!! and could not live a normal life!!!!Dr. Suher is a highly educated pleasant woman who believes in natural alternative solutions for all human health problems and she together with her big family got beautiful results after they used natural formulas for different disorders!!!! She sent me an email when I was on my way from Amman to Chicago informing me about the fast magic cure of her psoriasis after she used the natural cream IRIS PS (PSORIA TECH) CREAM together with **curcumin** for 8 weeks only!!!!!

She expressed to me about her pleasure and joy and said" It did work like a magic!!!!!" My severe psoriasis problem has been solved fast and I am able to live my normal life easily in less than 8 weeks!!!!!!"

A second story was told to me by one of my students; she was suffering from liver cirrhosis and ulcerative colitis and came to me with her mother asking about solution. She took the herbal capsules: LIV TECH, COLI TECH and CAMEL TECH together with **Curcumin**. She called me after 8 weeks only!!!She was shocked by the results; **all liver enzymes became almost normal** and she got other beautiful findings; **her colitis bleeding and diarrhea stopped completely and she could restore her normal life!!!!!**

Many other stories about using Turmeric Curcumin as an antioxidant anti-tumor immunity enhancing tool for different types of cancer!!

One of cancer patient is a medical doctor who suffered from colon cancer and liver and bone metastasis and his case was late. He started taking a natural immune therapy protocol: MG10, MG20, IMU TECH and CAMEL TECH together with **CURCUMIN** and a natural organic nutrition program for 6 month-course. Though we asked him to take a chemotherapy course from his doctor but he did refuse and his case now is fruitful and he was active in his clinic during the treatment course!!!!!

Huge number of people who got benefits of curcumin for acne, psoriasis, diabetes, gout, colon disorders, joint pain, weight loss, skin disorders and many other health problems!!!!

Modern science is beginning to recognize and understand the amazing healing qualities of turmeric and much research is currently being conducted.

Turmeric(the Latin name for turmeric is "Curcuma Longa", which comes from the **Arabic** name for the plant, "**Kurkum**) has been proven effective in treating some of the most intense ailments afflicting the world today including: Arthritis, Cancer, Alzheimer's Disease, Diabetes, Multiple Sclerosis, Atherosclerosis, HIV/AIDS, Sexually Transmitted Diseases (Hepatitis-C, Genital Herpes), Irritable Bowel Syndrome, Indigestion, Inflammation, Acne, Urinary Tract Infections, Kidney Infections, Gallstones, Anemia, Hemorrhoids, Liver Disease, Leprosy, Amenorrhea, Edema, Bronchitis, Common Cold, Headaches, Conjunctivitis, Bursitis, food poisoning, parasites, fever, diarrhea, poor circulation, lower back and abdominal pain. It can also be used as a mosquito repellent, wound healer, and immediate cure for scorpion stings. Turmeric helps balance the female reproductive and lactation systems, and in men it purifies and improves the health of semen. It is used to treat external ulcers that would not respond to other treatment 6, 8, 10 . Due to its vast array of medicinal purposes and versatility, turmeric is one of the most important herbs in any natural medicine cabinet.

I thank ALMIGHTY ALLAH for helping me learn the phytochemistry of herbs and computer to help people from many deadly health problems and I feel it is my responsibility to spread the science and experience among all people in the world.

Prof. Dr. Awad Mansour
Chicago, United States
March 2010

CURCUMIN AND ACNE

Major Causes of Acne

Acne is known to be partly hereditary. Several factors are known to be linked to acne:

Family/ Genetic history, Hormonal activity, such as menstrual cycles and puberty. Inflammation, skin irritation or scratching of any sort will activate inflammation. Stress. "increased acne severity" is "significantly associated with increased stress levels, Hyperactive sebaceous glands, Bacteria in the pores, Use of anabolic steroids, Exposure to certain chemical compounds. Chloracne is particularly linked to toxic exposure to dioxins, namely Chlorinated dioxins, chronic use of amphetamines or other similar drugs.

Sulfur is probably the oldest acne remedy known to medicine and its origins as an anti-acne treatment.

Some famous products in the market use **Benzoyl Peroxide** or **Salicylic acid** but both chemicals cause many side effects and skin irritation!!!!

Turmeric Curcumin(as a single herb or as a part of curry) serves both as an herb and a spice. It is a healing herb that is used effectively in different parts of the globe. While Indians use it for its anti-inflammatory properties, many other nations use this perennial herb for acne.

A teaspoon of **coriander juice**, mixed with a pinch of **turmeric powder**, is another effective home remedy for acne pimples and blackheads. The mixture should be applied to the face after thoroughly washing it every night. **Mint juice** can be used in a similar manner as coriander juice.

Natural Methods of Treating Acne:

You can find full details of the natural protocol of treating acne problems in our book: **How to Rid Acne in One Week without Medications** which will be printed in the United States.

We can draw the main guidelines of the protocol as follows:

1. **Juice that Heal:** Coriander juice (mixed with **turmeric** powder or mint juice) is used as a treatment for acne, applied to the face in the manner of toner.

2. **Food that Heal:** Lettuce, Cucumber, Curcumin are also helpful. Apple Cider Vinegar, Baking Powder are well known by their effects on improving acne.

3. **Herbs that Heal. Turmeric Curcumin,** Coriander, Aloe vera: Neem, Papaya and Calendula. *Propolis is one of the best herbs for acne.*

4. **Milk that Heals:** Camel milk (as narrated by Prophet Mohammad (PBUH) offers endless health benefits. One of those is treating acne. Patients who took 2 glasses of camel milk daily for 3 weeks found miracle results for acne!!!!!

5. **Herbal Tea that Heals:** Hundreds of acne cases who took a herbal tea composed of Lemon Balm, turmeric and coriander seed for 3 weeks could easily solve their acne without medications!!!!!

6. **Food Supplemnts that Heal:**, Vitamin B3, Zinc, MSM together with chlorophyll food supplement.

7. **Essential Oils that Heal:** Castor oil, Jojoba oil are cures for acne, turmeric oil is an excellent antiseptic. The relaxation oil: **Relax U:** was successfully used by acne patients!!!

8. **Soap that Heals: Nano Dead Sea Soap** was successfully used by hundreds who got rid of their acne in 2-3 weeks!!

9. **Cream that Heals:** Many acne patients used **Cellu Tech Cream** which is used for fatty cellulite got rid of their acne in 3-4 weeks.

10. **Bath that Heals:** Many patients cured their acne by using a 15-minute baking powder bath together with dead sea salt or mud!!!once daily for 3-4 weeks.

CURCUMIN AND ANEMIA

Anemia is a sign of few diseases and also diseases in itself. Anemia has been identified as a reduction of hemoglobin in the blood, which carries oxygen throughout the body. Anemia occurs when there is bleeding, when bone marrow cannot produce enough red blood cells, those produced have a defect, or when something interferes with the survival of red blood cells. Iron-deficiency anemia, caused by heavy or recurring bleeding, is the most prevalent form of the disorder. Persistent bleeding may occur from the digestive tract and is associated with diseases like gastritis, ulcerative colitis, hemorrhoids, hematuria (urine bleeding), inflammatory bowel disease, including leukemia and kidney disease, can produce anemia. Some types of anemia can be traced to genetic disorders. In children and adolescents, anemia can often be traced to insufficient dietary intake of iron. Loss of blood in menstruation is typically the cause of anemia among girls and women. In men, chronic occult bleeding in the gastrointestinal tract often leads to iron deficiency anemia. Signs and symptoms of anemia include fatigue, pallor, irritability, loss of appetite, backaches, headaches, soreness in the mouth and breathlessness. The homeopathic science suggests that deficiency should have to be corrected by necessary dietetic supplements.

Eating foods that contain adequate, easily absorbed sources of iron may be the best policy for anemia prevention. A balance diet that provides the Recommended Daily Allowance of iron is generally sufficient to guard against anemia. Certain chemicals interfere with iron absorption, for example, tannin in tea, polyphenols in coffee, and cadmium in cigarettes. Avoid these items those interfere iron absorption. Other important nutrients are **folic acid**, used by bone marrow to produce blood, and **vitamin B12**. Your diet should contain the following beverages in order to prevent Anemia:

Turmeric Curcumin is an excellent source of iron which directly helps curing anemia according to recent research.

The iron content in turmeric could prevent blood loss from excess bleeding.

From the phytochemical composition of Turmeric Curcumin we can notice a number of chemical compounds forming turmeric act as excellent source of iron, which clearly means that turmeric is a good candidate to be safely used to help for anemia!!!.

Turmeric Curcumin serves both as an herb and a spice. It is a healing herb that is used effectively in different parts of the globe. While Indians use it for its anti-inflammatory properties, many other nations use this herb for anemia.

We heared about many successful stories about using **curcumin** for anemia!!

Natural Methods of Treating Anemia:

You can find full details of a natural protocol of treating anemia problems in our book:

How to Fix Your Anemia in One Week withoutMedications which will be printed in the United States.

We can draw the main guidelines of the protocol as follows:

1. Juice that Heal: Wheatgrass, Grape, Beet and Black Currant juice can be very helpful.

2. Food that Heal: Sweet Potato, Beet, and Tomato are also helpful. Black Seed and Fenugreek are useful to solve anemia problem by the scientific research.

3. Herbs that Heal: Eating 1 tsp of alfalfa seed, fenugreek, curry(Curcumin)and black seed every morning for 3 months is good for anemia.

THE 50 MIRACLE CURES OF CURCUMIN

4. Milk that Heals: Camel milk (as narrated by Prophet Mohammad (PBUH) offers endless health benefits. One of those is treating anemia problems. My patients who took 2 glasses of camel milk daily with black seed for 3 months found miracle results for both anemia and sex!!!!!

5. Herbal Tea that Heals: Hundreds of anemia cases who took the herbal tea ;**Circu Tech Tea** which is simply composed of Nettle, Wormwood, Black Currant, Alfalfa, Curcumin and Coriander seed for 3-6 months could easily solve their anemia problem without medications!!!!!

6. Food Supplements that Heal: Many patients obtained excellent results by using the food supplement named: **Circu Tech** which contains a number of **iron-rich** herbs including curcumin!!Together with **chlorophyll, folic acid and Vitamin B12** food supplements.

CURCUMIN AND ARTHRITIS

Arthritis is inflammation of one or more joints, which results in pain, swelling, stiffness, and limited movement. There are over 100 different types of arthritis.

Symptoms

If you have arthritis, you may experience:

Joint pain, joint swelling, reduced ability to move the joint, redness of the skin around a joint, stiffness, especially in the morning, warmth around a joint.

From the phytochemical composition of turmeric we can notice a number of chemical compounds forming turmeric ;especially curcumin act as excellent anti-arthritic agent, which clearly means that turmeric is a good candidate to be safely used for arthritis, rheumatism, joint and back pain!!!.

Turmeric curcumin serves both as an herb and a spice. It is a healing herb that is used effectively in different parts of the globe. Indians use it and its oil for its anti-inflammatory properties, arthritis back pain, joints pain and gout.

The therapeutic properties of turmeric curcumin essential oil are as an **analgesic**, aphrodisiac, antispasmodic, carminative, depurative, deodorant, digestive, carminative, fungicidal, lipolytic, revitalizing, stimulant and stomachic. Turmeric oil can be useful to refresh and awake the mind. It can help for mental fatigue, migraine pain, tension and nervous weakness. **Turmeric oil's** warming effect is also helpful for alleviating pain such as **rheumatism, arthritis and muscle spasms**. There are some indications that are also can be useful in combating colds and flu.

Many stories successfully used turmeric curcumin as an anti-arthritis together with the food supplements **Rheuma Tech and Joint Tech** without any medications!!!!! One story was told to me by a lady from Emirates; she was suffering from back and joint pains and called me asking about solution. I asked her to take coriander tea for 4 weeks together with Curcumin. She called me after 3 weeks only!!!She was shocked by the results; all pains disappeared from the whole body and she got other beautiful findings; **she lost some of her extra weight!!!!!**

Natural Methods of Treating Arthritis Problems

You can find full details of the natural protocol of treating arthritis problems in our book:

How to Rid Arthritis without Medications which will be printed in the United States.

We can draw the main guidelines of the protocol as follows:

1. Juice that Heal: Cranberry and Celery juice can be very helpful.

2. Food that Heal: Cherry, Lettuce, Cucumber, Cabbage and Tomato are also helpful. Pomegranate, Ginger, Almonds and Walnuts and Grape Seed Extract, Baking Powder is well known by their effects on reducing arthritis and joints pain.

3. Herbs that Heal: Eating 1 tsp of alfalfa seed, curcumin, cinnamon, ginger with honey every morning for 3 months is good for arthritis. The Indian herb; Shilajit is one of the best herbs for arthritis.

4. Milk that Heals: Camel milk (as narrated by Prophet Mohammad (PBUH) offers endless health benefits. One of those is treating arthritis problems. Our patients who took 2 glasses of camel milk daily or the food supplements Rheuma Tech and Joint Tech for 3 months found miracle results for both arthritis and sex!!!!!

THE 50 MIRACLE CURES OF CURCUMIN

5. Herbal Tea that Heals: Hundreds of arthritis cases who took the herbal tea ;Uri Tech Tea which is simply composed of Celery, Alfalfa, Parsley, Curcumin and Coriander seed for 3-6 months could easily solve their arthritis problem without medications!!!!!

6. Food Supplemnts that Heal: Many patients obtained excellent results by using the food supplements named: Rheuma Tech and Joint Tech. Both contain a number of anti-arthritic herbs including **turmeric curcumin!!!!**

7. Essential Oils that Heal: A number of patients informed me about excellent results on their arthritic joints, back and knees by using a mix of turmeric oil and mustard oil for 6 weeks only!!! Turmeric oil stimulates circulation. Eases muscular stiffness, relieves arthritis and inflammatory conditions.

CURCUMIN AND BLADDER INFECTION

Bladder Infection (BI) is an infection by the bacteria of the urinary tract which includes kidney, uterus, bladder or urethra. The infection of the bladder can develop into cystitis- a very common problem faced by women. Bladder Infection can infect anyone but women are more susceptible to this disease. Children suffer from this disorder too but the headcount is very low in comparison to adults. Sexual intercourse is another reason for Bladder Infection.

From the phytochemical composition of turmeric we can notice a number of chemical compounds forming turmeric act as excellent anti-inflammatory agents, which clearly means that turmeric curcumin is a good candidate to be safely used for Bladder Infection!!!.

Turmeric curcumin serves both as an herb and a spice. It is a healing herb that is used effectively in different parts of the globe. While Indians use it for its anti-inflammatory properties, and hence for Bladder Infection.

Researchers have demonstrated that curcumin inhibited the growth and promoted cell death in three different melanoma cell lines. Curcumin appears to work by suppressing the production of the proteins in the cancer cells that normally protect the cells from cell death. All doses tested decreased cancer cell growth and triggered cell death. Higher doses were more effective, and the higher the dose used, the more cancer cells died according to the researchers findings.

Curcumin triggered the death of head and neck squamous cell carcinoma in a recent study published in Clinical Cancer Research. This research indicated that the addition of curcumin to cultures of squamous cell carcinoma in bladder resulted in a dose-dependent growth inhibition of three cell lines. Researchers also conducted in vivo studies with squamous cell tumors in mice. Topical application of curcumin also inhibited the growth of the cancer cells.

The usual protective measures recommended against UTI are clean personal habits and the use of supplements such as cranberry juice or the tannins found in cranberries and blueberries.drinking lots of clean water also helps in flushing out the system. Water also helps in flushing out the system.

Bladder infection and turmeric go hand in hand, and can really help to get rid of this infection, and more interestingly, help to stop it from coming back.

The Connection Between Curcumin and Hematuria

Curcumin has many beneficial properties, and acts as an anti-inflammatory, antioxidant, and antiviral. It can relieve swelling, and also serves to reduce the formation of blood clots.

In cases of hematuria where there is no serious underlying health condition causing blood to appear in the urine, curcumin has proven to be effective in relieving the symptoms. If the hematuria is being caused by a virus, curcumin can act as an antiviral agent to treat the virus itself.

Many conditions can be reduced or even prevented with curcumin and hematuria is one of them. However, if there is a disease or other health problem causing the hematuria, curcumin alone will not eliminate the causes. It's always best to see your doctor and ask for advice before trying to treat a health issue alone.

Many stories about using turmeric curcumin an anti-inflammatory tool for Bladder Infection!!!! Many Qatari and Saudi BI patients; got rid of it within 4 weeks only!!!!After starting taking coriander

THE 50 MIRACLE CURES OF CURCUMIN

tea, turmeric curcumin together with our food supplement **URI TECH** and **Cranberry Juice** without any medications!!!

Natural Methods of Treating Bladder Infection Problems:

You can find full details of a natural protocol of treating Bladder Infection problems in our book:

How to Rid Bladder Infection in 3 Weeks without Medications which will be printed in the United States.

We can draw the main guidelines of our protocol as follows:

1. Juice that Heals: Cranberry and drinking 2-3 glasses water on empty stomach can be very helpful.

2. Food that Heals: Lettuce, Cucumber, Cabbage are also helpful. Pomegranate, Baking Powder is well known by their effects on improving Bladder Infection.

3. Herbs that Heal: Eating 1 tsp of curcumin and cinnamon with honey every morning for 3 weeks is good for Bladder Infection. The Indian herb; Shilajit is one of the best herbs for BI._Dandelion and Tribulus terrestris are also useful.

4. Milk that Heals: Camel milk (as narrated by Prophet Mohammad (PBUH) offers endless health benefits. One of those is treating BI problems. My patients who took 2 glasses of camel milk daily with the food supplement Uri Tech for 3 months found miracle results for both BI and sex!!!!!

5. Herbal Tea that Heals: Hundreds of gout cases who took the herbal tea; Uri Tech Tea which is simply composed of Corn Silk, Parsley, turmeric curcumin and Coriander seed for 3-6 weeks could easily solve their Bladder Infection problem without medications!!!

6. Food Supplemnts that Heal: Many patients obtained excellent results by using the food supplement named: Uri Tech which contains a number of diuretic and anti-inflammatory herbs including

Turmeric Curcumin and Coriander seed!!!! together with chlorophyll supplement.

7. **Essential Oils that Heal:** You can make an essential oil by using equal parts of Coriander, sandalwood, frankincense, turmeric and juniper. Mix all these ingredients to make an oil to be rubbed over your bladder area. Continue this massaging technique for three to four days once the symptoms subside.

8. **Avoid irritant foods**: A diet which consists of processed food like cheese, chocolate, dairy products should be avoided. You should also avoid spicy food, caffeine, alcohol and cigarettes which otherwise is also harmful. Avoid carbonated drinks like beer, soda or any other drink with fizz, and Aspartame which is one of the artificial sweeteners.

CURCUMIN AND BODY ODOR & BAD BREATH

Body odor can be unpleasant as well as embarrassing, and for some people, it is a constant worry. The smell of waste products excreted by our bodies is also affected by toxins we have ingested or absorbed into our bodies. In a modern environment, our bodies are subjected to a host of chemicals and toxins in our food - including pollution in the air and even household cleaning products. Alcohol and tobacco is known to contribute to bad body odor – so try to cut back or avoid smoking and drinking completely.

Curcumin is widely used to cure halitosis and bad breath in general.

Turmeric Oil is a good deodorant too. It clears bad breath and eliminates mouth and body odor, when used internally or externally. When consumed or ingested, the typical aroma of this oil mixes with the sweat and fights body odor as well as fights oral odor as its scent, coming up from your stomach, fills your mouth. This also helps inhibit the bacterial growth in mouth and around sweat glands and thereby fighting odor. Mixed in water, when externally applied or used as a mouthwash, it again does it all!!!

Turmeric Oil cleans blood of toxins and thus acts as a detoxifier or blood purifies. It helps remove the regular toxins like uric acid, heavy metals and certain compounds and hormones produced by the body itself, from blood, as well as other foreign toxins which get into blood accidentally.

There are a number of other home remedies to rid bad odors from mouth and body such as:

Chlorophyll: To prevent body odor, drink a glass of water in the morning, on an empty stomach, along with 500 mg wheat grass. The chlorophyll present in the grass will help in reducing body and mouth odor.

Mint

Parsley

Green and Black Tea

Milk Thistle is very famous to remove toxins from the liver.

Zinc is also very beneficial for curing bad breath.

There are many herbs also which helps to remove the bad odor like rosemary, parsley. Spearmint and tarragon, these herbs help to freshen up your mouth.

Also make a solution of baking soda by adding water and do regular gargles from this solution. It can also clean the tongue. This is one of the excellent home based remedy to reduce the bad breath. You can also apply baking soda to your armpits as well as to your feet, to reduce body odor.

While bathing, add white vinegar or apple cider vinegar to a mug of water and use it to rinse the armpits. This will definitely help in lessening the body odor.

Mix 10 drops of the essential oil such as turmeric oil, Lavender or Bergamot oil in 30 ml water. Apply this mixture on the armpits to reduce body odor.

CURCUMIN AND CANCER

Curcumin is indigenous to southern Europe, but it is used widely in Asiatic and South American cuisine as well as that of the Mediterranean region.

Curcumin's anti-tumorigenic properties have been demonstrated in relation to colon, pancreatic, prostate, skin and breast cancer.It works by protecting against the damaging effects of lipid oxidation associated with this malignancy. It is highly probable that curcumin also contributes to the low incidences of several other cancer types seen in the populations of Eastern nations that consume large quantities of this spice.

Curcumin Helps Fight Breast and Liver Cancers and Many Other Types of Cancer

Curcumin possesses several anti-cancer benefits that make it highly effective as a cancer preventive agent against almost any type of cancer. One of its most talked-about features is its antioxidant action.

From Extension Life Magazine it is reported:

Curcumin enhances immunity

Curcumin can also help the body fight off cancer should some cells escape apoptosis. When researchers looked at the lining of the intestine after ingestion of curcumin, they found that CD4+ T-helper and B type immune cells were greater in number. In addition to this localized immune stimulation, curcumin also enhances immunity in general. Researchers in India have documented increased antibodies and more immune action in mice given Curcumin was noticed.

Curcumin stops angiogenesis

All of the above actions of curcumin stop cancer before it has a chance to become detectable. If cancer grows to the point that it is a detectable tumor, curcumin can still have an effect.

Certain enzymes enable tumors to create a blood supply for themselves. Known as "angiogenesis, " this phenomenon allows tumors to invade surrounding tissue and spread. Working with blood vessels of the eye (where angiogenesis creates big problems for vision), researchers at Tufts University were able to inhibit blood vessel formation by using curcuminoids. Curcumin blocks AP-1, which enhances angiogenesis.

Curcumin may also inhibit angiogenesis by chelating metals used by enzymes that promote the growth of blood vessels. Some of the enzymes as Metalloproteinases require metals to work. Curcumin chelates iron and probably copper-both of which help metal loproteinases create new blood vessels for tumors. In a study on a highly invasive form of human liver cancer, curcumin inhibited metastasis 70% by suppressing metalloproteinase-9. Curcumin appears to be very protective against liver cancer. In a more recent study, the incidence of liver cancer was slashed 62%, with the number of tumors decreasing by 81% in mice given curcumin four days before a carcinogenic chemical.

The cancer preventive effects of curcumin are powerful and proven. Curcumin interferes with the ability of estrogen-mimicking and other chemicals to do damage (a trait it shares with I3C). It is a powerful antioxidant that can alter gene expression, stop the cell cycle, and induce the self-destruction of cancer cells without affecting healthy ones. By blocking signals known as kinases, curcumin interrupts signals that enable cancer cells to grow. In addition, curcumin enhances immunity and blocks the invasion and metastases of tumors. Curcumin significantly reduces the risk of cancer after chemical exposure, and appears especially beneficial against colon and liver cancers. The actions of curcumin have been

THE 50 MIRACLE CURES OF CURCUMIN

the subject of presentations at major meetings on cancer research, and the object of study by researchers at the most prestigious universities in the world. **If curcumin were a drug, it would be hailed as one of the best all-around cancer drugs ever invented.** As it is, it's a phytochemical with impeccable credentials, thousands of years of use behind it, and a very small price tag. **No wonder a host of drug companies want to imitate it.**

Curcumin kills cancer cells

Curcumin can stop cancer in its earliest stages, long before it's detectable. It works at the level of the cell. One of the things it does is to tell damaged cells to self-destruct so they won't keep multiplying. The process is called "apoptosis" and it's the body's way of destroying abnormal cells that can become cancerous. Cancer cells can circumvent the process, but curcumin can override them and send "self-destruct" signals to many different types of cancer cells. **Curcumin does not induce apoptosis of healthy cells, only cancerous ones.** It identifies cancer cells by their abnormal chemistry. Indian researchers findings, published in the Journal of Biological Chemistry, may lead to ways of making most types of cancer susceptible to curcumin's effects.

Before apoptosis is induced, curcumin stops cancer cells from multiplying. In cancer research, this is known as "interrupting the cell cycle." The cell cycle can be interrupted at several different points. This is the rationale behind using various chemotherapy treatments in one person. One drug stops the cells when they are in one stage of growth; another stops them at another stage. Using a variety of drugs that stop growth at different stages increases the chances of killing all the cancer cells. Curcumin arrests the growth of cancer cells in the G2 stage.

Other phytochemicals stop the cell cycle at other stages. Genistein, a soy phytochemical, arrests growth at G2, like curcumin. But

(EGCG) from **green tea**, arrests cancer cell growth at the G1 phase. *Combining EGCG with curcumin increases the odds of killing more cells.* Researchers at Sloan-Kettering Cancer Center have suggested that EGCG and curcumin be used together for cancer prevention.

Drug companies rush to make synthetic versions

One of the hottest areas of oncology drug development is in the area of kinase inhibitors. Kinases are the equivalent of phone lines into cancer cells. There are over 2000 known protein kinases, or phone lines. These lines run from the outside of a cell into the DNA command center. They carry messages. Cut these lines, and you can effectively stop the growth of some types of cancer cells.

Curcumin effectively blocks some of the lines. In cells treated with curcumin, certain "grow" signals are blocked from reaching the cell.

The most well-studied growth factor blocked by curcumin is nuclear factor-k B. NF-kB is activated by chemical messengers known as cytokines. Cytokines help the immune system, but they also activate signals that tell cells to multiply, grow. By interfering with those signals, curcumin effectively stops the growth of cancer cells by kinase pathways. It has been demonstrated, for example, that curcumin can prevent the bug that causes ulcers (*Helicobacter pylori*) from causing cancer. *H. pylori* increases levels of a cytokine (IL-8) that activates NF-kB. Curcumin blocks the process.

One of the things that sets curcumin apart from most other anti-cancer supplements (I3C being an exception), is that this phenolic can actually block chemicals from getting inside cells. Importantly, curcumin can interfere with pesticides that mimic estrogen. These include DDT and dioxin, two extremely toxic chemicals that contaminate America's water and food. (Dioxin is so toxic that a

THE 50 MIRACLE CURES OF CURCUMIN

few ounces of it could wipe out the entire population of New York City). Curcumin has the unique ability to fit through a cellular doorway known as the aryl hydrocarbon receptor. This is a feat it shares with estrogen and estrogen-mimicking chemicals. Because it can compete for the same doorway, curcumin has the power to block access to the cell and protect against estrogen mimickers.

Like estrogen, estrogen-mimicking chemicals promote the growth of breast cancer. In a study on human breast cancer cells, curcumin reversed growth caused by 17b-estradiol by 98%. DDT's growth-enhancing effects on breast cancer were blocked about 75% by curcumin.

Two other estrogen mimickers were tested for their ability to enhance breast cancer. Chlordane and endosulfane together make breast cancer cells grow about as much as17b-estradiol. Curcumin can reverse that growth about 90%. Adding the soy phytochemical, genistein, causes a 100% growth arrest.

Curcumin's ability to block other chemicals have been documented. It has been tested against paraquat (weed killer), nitrosamines (in cooked meat and "lunch" meats) and carbon tetrachloride (a solvent in varnish and other products). In all cases, curcumin is able to block the chemical's effect. The beneficial effects are evident in a study where mice were treated with diethylnitrosamine. All mice treated with this chemical would usually develop liver cancer. However, when treated with curcumin, the percentage of animals developing cancer went from 100% to 38%, and the number of tumors dropped by 81%.

Drug companies are rushing to patent chemicals that do what curcumin does-inhibit kinases. AstraZeneca has gotten one off the ground called "Iressa". Iressa inhibits protein kinase C (PKC), a kinase that plays a significant role in cancer. PKC transmits signals from the "epidermal growth factor (EGF) receptor." Cutting off signal transmission through EGF significantly slows the growth of any cancer that uses this factor to grow-glioma, breast, prostate, skin and lung cancers.

Curcumin has long been known for its ability to prevent skin cancer. In 1993, researchers in Taiwan reported that curcumin inhibits PKC. The next year it was reported that curcumin blocks EGF signals up to 90% and stops growth.

It turns out that the structure of curcumin enables it to inhibit multiple kinases. This ability is shared with other phytochemicals including silymarin, apigenin and hypericin. While drug companies rush to try to recreate safe, patentable, chemical versions of this structure, curcumin sits ready and available for use. Blocking kinases, however, is only one of curcumin's anti-cancer effects.

Nano-capsule to boost person's absorption of curcumin

WASHINGTON - A nano-sized capsule being developed by researchers boosts the person's uptake of curcumin, the main ingredient in tumeric powder, and can be used in treatment of several diseases including colon cancer and Alzheimer's.

Clinical trials are checking its safety and effectiveness for colon cancer, psoriasis, and Alzheimer's disease. However, digestive juice in the gastrointestinal tract quickly destroys curcumin so that little actually gets into the blood. Koji Wada and colleagues note that curcumin is a potent anti-oxidant found in turmeric. Scientists have known for years that encapsulating insulin and certain other drugs into structures called liposomes can boost absorption.

The scientists prepared the liposomes encapsulating curcumin and fed them to lab rats, says a release of the American Chemcial

Society (ACS). Encapsulating more than quadrupled absorption of curcumin, and also boosted antioxidant levels in the blood.

The encapsulating process could be an answer to the problem of increasing curcumin's absorption in the digestive environment of the gastrointestinal tract, they suggest.

Nanocurcumin prepared by a team of researchers at School of Medicine, Baltimore, Maryland provides an opportunity to expand the clinical reports of this efficacious agent by enabling ready aqueous dispersion. Future studies utilizing nanocurcumin are warranted in pre-clinical *in vivo* models of cancer and other diseases that might benefit from the effects of curcumin.

Other researchers at Harvard School Used Gold-Citrate Nanoparticles and Curcumin Nanomedicine to Target Cancer at a Single Cell Level.

Curcumin encased in nanoparticles has been found highly effective in treating breast cancers. Researchers at the M D Anderson Cancer Center in the University of Texas, US, fabricated the nanoparticles using silk fibre rich in keratin (silk fibroin) and chitosan (a polysaccharide) polymers. The team found the breast cancer cells absorbed nanocurcumin very well. The results suggested nanocurcumin would be able to treat breast cancer but further studies are needed. The results were published in the May 2009 issue of the *International Journal of Nanomedicine*.

CURCUMIN AND CELLULITE

Mix base oil with **curcumin**, thyme, and wintergreen or carrot essential oils and use to massage the cellulite affected area.

Diane Irons, author of Teen Beauty Secrets suggests rubbing warm coffee grounds into the fatty area.

Diane Irons also suggests rubbing down the body with Epson salts while in the shower to help with the cellulite.

It is suggested to use our cellulite oil and cream: *Cellu Tech Oil and Cream* which include **curcumin**, green tea extract and Lemon oil with strong massage to get excellent results.

From: sparkpeople.com: Lose inches & cellulite DIY Body Wrap and more Body wrapping is a therapeutic treatment that is used to detoxify the body using simple all natural ingredients. These simple readily available ingredients have been used over the years traditionally to tighten and tone the skin and help stimulate the body to rid itself of trapped toxins, excess fat and excessive trapped lymph fluids. This detoxification improves the appearance of cellulite, creates inch loss, and helps tighten and tone the skin.

HERBAL BODY WRAP RECIPE

Mix a cup of 369 corn oil with 1/2 cup of grapefruit juice and 2 teaspoons dried thyme. Massage into hip, thigh, and buttock areas. Cover with plastic wrap to lock in body heat.

(*For extra results lay a heating pad over each area for five minutes*).

CLAY BODY WRAP RECIPE

1 cup bentonite or green clay
1/4 cup sea salt
2 tbsp. olive oil
2 cups water

Boil water and add sea salt until it is dissolved. Add remaining ingredients and stir. Adjust the water if necessary to form a wet

paste. Rub the mixture over your entire body and cover yourself with thin towels or a clean white sheet. Most salons will recommend that you use proper wrapping sheets as the compaction helps to squeeze the tissues together for greater results.
Lay in the tub for a minimum of 45 min. to one hour.
Cellulite and Fat Fighting Ingredient Tips Coffee Grounds: Rub coffee grounds on cellulite/fat area before taking a shower every night. The coffee helps firm the area and lessen that "cheese" look. *WHY?*

Caffeine is the first ingredient in most cellulite treatments. The same way caffeine gets us moving in the morning, it can also help to get our fat cells moving. This trick, employed by famous models and beauty contestants, involves rubbing warm coffee grounds into the cellulite-laden areas of your legs, using your hands or a loofah mitt. To intensify the treatment, take a rolling pin and roll the area to further smooth out the cellulite.

Another Important Anti-Cellulite Tools:

In ***MAGIC TOUCH CENTERS IN CHICAGO, AMMAN AND EMIRATES*** they use together with our anti-cellulite oils, creams and loofah-built–in Dead Sea soap and nano soap: Nano-Scrubbers, Nano Steam, Acoustic Massagers.

Instant results are obtained within a week!!!!

Drink Green Tea Daily: WHY?

According to research published in the American Journal of Clinical Nutrition "consumption of green tea produces thermogenesis and increases energy expenditure and fat oxidation in humans.

Green tea is an active ingredient used in many of the top weight loss products. When a weight loss product claims it contains natural ingredients, green tea is nearly always in the list. Did you know that?

Essential Oils for fighting Cellulite and Fat:

Buy essential oils (they are cheap on Ebay) and use them for a massage every day. If you hate the feel of oil, try adding the oils in a cream which you use as your moisturizer.

WHY?

The "bumps" of cellulite are composed of fat, cellular wastes and water. The oils used to counteract the condition improve circulation, strengthen connective tissues, encourage the elimination of wastes and fight fluid retention.

Experiment with the following oils: (Always use a carrier oil) . Defeat your cellulite and fatty areas with:

Basil, birch, cedar wood, clary sage, coriander, turmeric, cypress, fennel, geranium, ginger, grapefruit, juniper, lemon, orange, patchouli, pine, rosemary, and thyme oils.

Always keep in mind, the essential oils need to be mixed with a carrier oil*. It is very dangerous to use essential oils on their own on your skin without mixing them with carrier oil. Please use caution *.Examples of carrier oils are sweet almond, apricot kernel, grape seed, avocado, peanut, olive, pecan, macadamia nut, sesame, evening primrose, walnut and wheat germ.*

Special Cellulite Massaging Oil:
5 drops fennel oil
4 drops rosemary oil
2 drops coriander oil
4 drops lavender oil
Add these oils in 20 ml of carrier oil. Massage into affected area daily.

Moisturizer Cellulite Rub:
2 drops bay oil
2 drops lemon oil
4 drops lavender oil
Add these oils in 20 ml of sesame oil. Massage into affected area daily.

Add Algae Powder to any of your favorite body lotion/ cream. This combination will help reduce cellulite and water retention and it also aids in the reduction of toxins and stress.

Adding 2 tablespoons of this powder to your bath will leave both your body and mind free of impurities.

Cellulite Oils/Herbs: White Birch, Cypress, Sweet Fennel, Geranium, Grapefruit, Juniper, Lemon, Parsley, Rosemary, Thyme, Coriander and Turmeric.

A NEW ANTI-CELLULITE SOAP FROM DEAD SEA

IRIS the Dead Sea Natural Cosmetics Company in Jordan has manufactured a miracle anti-cellulite Nano Soap from Vegetable Glycerine, Dead Sea Mud, Coffee, Curcumin, Green Tea, and Lavender Oil .This miracle soap(available at **Magic Touch Centers** *branches)works as: Excellent Instant Desinfictant, Fast Anti-Cellulite Soap, Natural Whitening Agent and a Fast Anti-Acne and Anti-Wrinkle Agent.*

CURCUMIN AND CHOLESTEROL

Cholesterol is a fatty substance, also called a lipid, that's produced by the liver. It's also found in foods high in saturated fat, like fatty meats, egg yolks, shellfish, and whole-milk dairy products. It's a vital part of the structure and functioning of our cells. However, high levels of cholesterol in your blood may lead to the slow buildup of plaque in the arteries over time, a serious disease called atherosclerosis.

The fact is that cholesterol can be harmful to your health when there's too much cholesterol in your blood. Whether you have high cholesterol may depend on your lifestyle. Eating a lot of fats and not getting enough exercise can cause cholesterol levels to rise. Cholesterol is also, in part, a result of your genetic makeup.

Everyone with high cholesterol needs to keep it under control, but it may be even more important for some groups of people, such as

- People with a family history of early heart disease
- People with high blood pressure
- People with diabetes
- People with obesity
- People with continuous stress
- Males over age 45
- Females over age 55
- Smokers

From the phytochemical composition of turmeric we can notice a number of chemical compounds forming turmeric act as anti-lipid and anti-cholesterol agents, which clearly means that turmeric is a good candidate to be safely used for high cholesterol.

Turmeric serves both as an herb and a spice. It is a healing herb that is used effectively in different parts of the globe. While Indians use it for its anti-inflammatory properties, many other nations use this perennial herb for high cholesterol.

For high cholesterol management it has been shown that turmeric curcumin acts as an anti-lipid agent and also helps in the vasodilation of veins!!

Many high cholesterol cases used turmeric curcumin from kitchen together with the powerful Choles Tech food supplement and after 3 months they got excellent results without any medications!!!!!

Natural Methods of Treating High Cholesterol:

You can find full details of a natural protocol of treating high cholesterol in our book:

How to Lower Your High Cholesterol to Normal without Medications which will be printed in the United States.

We can draw the main guidelines of our protocol as follows:

1. Juice that Heal: Acai, Tomato, Cucumber, and Celery juice can be helpful.

2. Food that Heal: Dark Chocolate, Peanut Butter, Lettuce, Cucumber, Sunflower seeds, Yogurt and Tomato are also helpful. Garlic is useful to lower the blood high cholesterol by the scientific research. Apple cider vinegar: It is said that an 8oz.apple juice with a tablespoon of apple cider vinegar will lower cholesterol. Almonds and Walnuts are very famous for lowering cholesterol. Grape Seed Extract and Pomegranate are well known by their effect in lowering cholesterol.

3. Herbs that Heal: Eating 1 tsp of flax seed, curcumin and black seed every morning for 3 months is said to prevent high cholesterol due to heredity factors. They also lower high cholesterol due to obesity, as both seeds have weight reducing properties. The Indian famous herb; Guggul is very famous for this purpose.

THE 50 MIRACLE CURES OF CURCUMIN

4. Milk that Heals: Camel milk (as narrated by Prophet Mohammad (PBUH) offers endless health benefits. One of those is treating high cholesterol. Camel milk is said to be the vasodilator of the Future". My patients who took 2 glasses of camel milk daily or our food supplement: CholesTech for 3 months found miracle results for both high cholesterol and sex!!!!!

5. Herbal Tea that Heals: Hundreds of high cholesterol cases who took the herbal tea ;Heart & Love Tea which is simply composed of Cinnamon, Turmeric, Fenugreek and Coriander seed for 3-6 months could easily reduce their high cholesterol to normal without medications!!!!!

6. Food Supplements that Heal: Many patients obtained excellent results by using the food supplement named: Choles Tech which contains a number of anti-lipid herbs including turmeric curcumin!!!!

7. Essential Oils that Heal: The oil mix which includes turmeric oil in it was successfully used with hundreds of high cholesterol patients together with coriander tea and all of them became high cholesterol free!!!!!!

Curcumin shares some of the same effects on the liver as silymarin and cynarin. It has demonstrated similar liver protection activity to silymarin. Curcumin is believed to also be converted to a choleretic compound, perhaps even caffeic acid. Curcumin's documented choleretic effects support its historical use in treating liver and gallbladder disorders. Like cynara extracts, curcumin has also been shown to lower cholesterol levels .

A recent experiment from the Central Food Research Center, in India, studied the effects of Turmeric Curcumin mixed with Red Pepper Capsaicin on rats that had been fed a very high-fat, high-cholesterol diet. Researchers saw significant drops in total cholesterol(up to 22%)and triglyceride levels in the rats as cholesterol was broken down faster and eliminated.

Animal studies have shown that turmeric lowers cholesterol levels and inhibits the oxidation of LDL ("bad cholesterol", responsible for clogging of arteries). When LDL becomes oxidized, it creates deposits in the walls of blood vessels and contributes to the formation of arteriosclerosis. Turmeric may also prevent platelet buildup along the walls of injured blood vessels, another common cause of blood clots and artery blockage that can result in heart attacks and strokes.

It is important to know that researchers discovered that high cholesterol is not responsible for arteries blockage. Chlamydia Pneumoniae is accused to cause this problem!!!!!! *James* **Phillips** (*JAMA.* 1999;282:2071-2073)*mentioned that: Recent studies have shown an association between an obligate intracellular bacterium, Chlamydia pneumoniae, and atherosclerosis.*

CURCUMIN AND CONSTIPATION

Here are the best 12 herbal remedies for Constipation (see carihal.com):

12 Top and Best Constipation Herbal Remedies:

Constipation refers to a health condition when fewer bowel movements are occurred than it should be. It is indeed an uncomfortable and embarrassing health situation that even require serious medical attention if continues for longer period. Typically, if you are having less than three bowel movements in a week, quite obviously you are suffering from constipation problem. However, lack of exercise and unhealthy diet can contribute to constipation development. Constipation is not a serious problem till it becomes chronic.

However not so serious at initial stages, but it is always better that you should find ways for constipation cure and apply them accordingly as required. This article focuses on various types of constipation cure and their associated benefits.

1.Triphala Since ancient times, Triphala is well respected for its various nutritional benefits including a sophisticated solution as constipation cure. Triphala is an Indian preparation that constitutes three herbal components, namely, Amalaki, Haritaki and Bibhitaki. Triphala serves the purpose of both purgative laxative as well as lubricating bulk laxative. So, if you are suffering from constipation problem, you can definitely count on Triphala as the best constipation cure. Triphala functions nicely even in the case of chronic constipation problem. It effectively cleanses the colon and digestive system. Hence it protects the body from harmful bodily wastages.

2. Psyllium husk This offers a special household solution to constipation cure. It is obtained from the seed of the Plantago ovata plant. In Ayurvedic literature, this herb has been illustrated as an emollient, fresh, gentle laxative and diuretic.

3. Bael Fruit: Bael fruit is truly popular for its ability to combat constipation. If you are suffering from constipation problem and would like to count on Bael fruit while looking for a cure to constipation, you need to use this fruit in its raw form regularly, for at least 2 to 3 months of time, prior to meals.

4. Senna: Identified in the name of Markandika in Ayurveda, Senna offers an ideal way to relieve constipation and encourage bowel movement smoothly.

5. Licorice: This is beneficial for softening the stools. Also it has nutritional value as it is rich in fiber content. It works very effectively if it is combined with Senna.

6. Coriander Leaves The primary function of this herb is to boost the digestive system.

7. Grapes Grapes are truly effective in treating constipation in addition to providing nutritional benefits. With its outstandingly delicious and sophisticated flavor, grapes offer an excellent solution for constipation treatment of both sorts, temporary and chronic.

8. Dandelion: To drink a tea mixed with dandelion powder can restore your health. This is not a mere saying, but in reality dandelion can offer you a miracle. It has the ability to promote bowel movement and offer you a relief from constipation problem.

9. Sweet Figs This is commonly used in the case of constipation. It has a traditional value. It is also effective in digestion problem.

10. Amaltas This is scientifically known as Cassia fistula. Its fruit is used, specifically the fruit pulp. You can mix the pulp with the lukewarm water and drink it on a regular basis. It will provide you a relief from constipation problem. It is also safe to use during

THE 50 MIRACLE CURES OF CURCUMIN

pregnancy, however, seeking medical attention is always recommended.

11. Honey. Honey offers several health benefits and protects us from many health hazards. This is also true in the case of constipation. If you mix one teaspoon of honey in one cup of warm water and drink it regularly in the morning before breakfast, you will certainly come out from your constipation problem.

12. PRUNE JUICE IS ONE OF THE BEST IN EAST AND WEST!!!!!

CURCUMIN AND DENGUE FEVER

Dengue is an acute infectious viral disease transmitted by the Aedes mosquitoes. Common in tropical climates, the dengue fever is also known as "break-bone fever" due to the severe joint and muscle pain suffered by the patients. Other symptoms of dengue include severe headache, fever, and intense joint pain, which will usually last about a week. The fever will usually subside after 2 to 5 days and thereafter will rise again followed by rashes on the skin. The dengue hemorrhagic fever is another form of the disease, which is more serious and can be fatal. More than 300, 000 patients in West Saudi are suffering from Dengue fever.

There is only one fast solution for Dengue fever which is MC10 herbal supplement.It was very effective in curing all Saudi cases in 24 hours. The same product is used for Malaria.

There is a famous coriander soup ; extensively used for Dengue fever:

CRAB SOUP

"Crab Soup", is a delicious soup and can be easily prepared. Believe me that after 3 servings of this crab soup, the patient's blood platelets will increase and fever will subside. Just give it a try.

Ingredients:

2 crabs which have been cleaned and cut into two (can be any type, for instance flower crab or tiger crab)

1 inch of ginger (cut into small pieces)

1 clove of garlic (crushed) or 1 tsp of curcumin

1 shallot (pounded)

Cooking oil (2 spoonful)

4 ounces of water

Salt

5 Peppercorns (pounded)

1 lemon grass (crushed)

Juice from 1 lime (squeezed)

1 strip each of coriander leaf and Chinese leak (cut into small pieces)

Directions:

Heat the cooking oil in a pot. Put in the shallot, garlic, ginger and peppercorn and fry (in low heat) until you can smell the sweet and tangy aroma.

Put in the crabs and flip the crabs occasionally until both sides turned red

Put in water and lemon grass

Turn the heat low and cover the pot with a lid. Bring the soup to boil for at least 15 minutes.

Put in the lime juice and some salt (as desired)

Stir the ingredients in the pot for 5 minutes

Put in the coriander leaf and Chinese leak on the dish

The soup is now ready to be served

CURCUMIN AND DIABETES

From the Appendix which discusses the phytochemical composition of turmeric we notice a number of compounds which are either anti-diabetic or hypoglycemic and in both cases turmeric lowers blood sugar if it is used as an herbal tea on daily basis.

Some other compounds of turmeric raise the good cholesterol; HDL, and lowers bad cholesterol; LDL which may cause or worsen diabetes!!!!

Turmeric serves both as an herb and a spice. It is a healing herb that is used effectively in different parts of the globe. While Indians use it for its anti-inflammatory properties, many European nations use this herb for its anti-diabetic qualities.

Hypoglycaemic activity: A 50% ethanolic extract of the rhizome produced a lowering of blood sugar (by 37.2% and 54.5% at 3 and 6 hours after administration) in alloxan-diabetic rats. When given together with Momordica charantia and Phyllanthus emblica (all in powder form), it exhibited an even more pronounced anti-diabetic action.

In diabetic rats, a 30% improvement in urine sugar and urine volume profiles was observed with feeding fenugreek seed mucilage and spent turmeric. Fasting blood glucose showed a 26% and 18% improvement with fenugreek seed and spent turmeric feeding to diabetic rats, respectively.

(From: Nutrition Research, Volume 25, Issue 11, Pages 1021-1028)

Main types of diabetes:

Type 1 ("insulin-dependent" and previously called "juvenile diabetes"). Type 1 diabetes is associated with a partial or total damage of beta cells in the pancreas which do not produce enough amounts of insulin. It develops most often in children and young adults. Type 1 diabetes represents 5%-10% of diabetics and is traditionally treated with insulin.

Type 2 ("insulin-independent" or sometimes called "adult-onset diabetes"). Type 2 diabetes is associated with insulin resistant cells. It is much more common and usually develops in older adults Type 2. diabetes represents 90-95% of diabetics.

Gestational (pregnancy-related). Some women develop diabetes during pregnancy. It affects 3 to 5 percent of all pregnant women. Although it goes away after pregnancy, these women have a higher chance for developing type 2 diabetes later in their lives.

Symptoms of Diabetes

Millions of people have diabetes and do not even know it because the symptoms develop so gradually, people often do not recognize them. Some people, particularly pre-diabetics, have no symptoms at all. Diabetics may have SOME or NONE of the following symptoms:

- Frequent urination
- Excessive thirst
- Extreme hunger
- Unexplained weight loss
- Sudden vision changes
- Numbness in hands or feet
- Poor blood circulation
- Poor sleep
- Feeling fatigue and tired most of the time
- Dry skin
- Sores that is slow to heal
- More infections than usual

Natural Methods of Treating Diabetes:

THE 50 MIRACLE CURES OF CURCUMIN

You can find full details of a natural protocol of treating diabetes in our book:

How to Lower Your Sugar from 400 to 100 without Medications which will be printed in the United States soon.

We can draw the main guidelines of our protocol as follows:

1. **Juice that Heal:** Wheatgrass, Tomato, Cucumber, Okra, Celery and Cabbage juice can be helpful.

2. **Food that Heal:** Lettuce, Cucumber, Yogurt and Tomato are also helpful... Garlic and Onion are useful to lower the blood sugar by the scientific research. Apple Cider Vinegar on green salad is daily recommended.

3. **Herbs that Heal:** Eating 1 tsp of curry leaves every morning for 3 months is said to prevent diabetes due to heredity factors. It also cures diabetes due to obesity, as the leaves have weight reducing properties. As the weight drops, the diabetic patients stop passing sugar in urine. **Turmeric** is one of the best spices that helps detoxify liver and lowers blood sugar!!!Propolis is one of the excellent products for lipid and diabetes(according to a study published in P. J. Pharm. Sci., Vol.22, No.2, April 2009, pp.168-174).

4. **Milk that Heals:** Camel milk (as narrated by Prophet Mohammad (PBUH) offers endless health benefits. One of those is treating diabetes. Camel milk is said to be the Insulin of the Future". My patients who took 2 glasses of camel milk daily or our food supplement: Camel Tech for 3 months found miracle results for both diabetes and sex!!!!!

5. **Herbal Tea that Heals:** Hundreds of diabetics who took our herbal tea ;Dia Tea which is simply composed of Fenugreek, Cinnamon and Turmeric for 3-6 months could easily reduce their blood sugar from 400 to 100 without medications!!!!!

6. Food Supplemnts that Heal: Many patients obtained excellent results by using the food supplement named: GlucoLife which contains a number of hypoglycemic herbs including Turmeric!!!!

7. Essential Oils that Heal:

Coriander oil for type II diabetes

Researchers from the University of Cairo used Coriander Oil together with other essential oils and experimented them on diabetic mice and they got excellent results!!!!!

CURCUMIN AND DIGESTION

For good digestion, Curcumin has a long and venerable history as a warming herb that stimulates the digestive tract. Its mild aromatic properties have been used for thousands of years to stop stomach irritation when taken at proper dosages. The exact mechanism is not entirely understood, but modern research confirms that the herb does protect gastric mucosa, helping to ease indigestion and other digestive problems. It is known to reduce intestinal gas formation and acts as a fine carminative, helping to expel intestinal gas. This warming herb is also thought to stimulate the appetite and is sometimes used to help those fighting anorexia.

Curcumin's main reputation lies with its ability to support the digestive system. It is a fine stomach tonic that stimulates the secretion of gastric juices thereby helping to promote good digestion. Curcumin is said to reduce irritation in the gastrointestinal tract, including heartburn (acid reflux), *nausea and stomach pain. Because Curcumin boosts the production of enzymes that digest sugar and fat, it is said to cut fat from the blood and Indian healers have used Turmeric for thousands of years in Ayurvedic medicine in weight loss regimens.*

Curcumin serves both as an herb and a spice. It is a healing herb that is used effectively in different parts of the globe. While Indians use it for its anti-inflammatory properties, many other nations use this herb for digestion.

We heared many successful stories about using **curcumin** for digestion!!

Natural Methods of Treating Digestion:

You can find full details of a natural protocol of treating digestion problems in our book:

How to Fix Indigestion in One Week without Medications which will be printed in the United States.

We can draw the main guidelines of our protocol as follows:

1. Juice that Heal: Wheatgrass, Mint-Lemon juice can be very helpful.

2. Food that Heal: Okra is also helpful. Propolis and Licorice are useful to solve digestion problems by the scientific research.

3. Herbs that Heal: Chamomile, Caraway, Fennel, Lemon Balm, Mint, Ginger are good for digestion.

4. Milk that Heals: Camel milk (as narrated by Prophet Mohammad (PBUH) offers endless health benefits. One of those is treating digestion problems. My patients who took 2 glasses of camel milk daily for 3 months found miracle results for both digestion and sex!!!!!

5. Herbal Tea that Heals: Hundreds of anemia cases who took the herbal tea; Diges Tech Tea which is simply composed of Mint, Chamomile, Ginger, Lemon Balm and Curcumin for 3 months could easily solve their digestion easily.

CURCUMIN AND DYSENTRY

Dysentery is not a disease but a symptom of a potentially deadly illness. The term refers to any case of infectious bloody diarrhea, a scourge that kills as many as 700, 000 people worldwide every year. People afflicted with amebic dysentery often suffer profuse, bloody diarrhea along with a fever, intense stomach pain, and rapid weight loss. Bacillary dysentery causes small, frequent stools mixed with blood and mucus. Cramps are common, and a patient may occasionally strain painfully, without success, to evacuate the bowels.

Curcumin is a valuable herb in treating digestive disorders. One or two teaspoons of curcumin, added to fresh buttermilk, is highly beneficial in treating indigestion, nausea, dysentery, hepatitis and ulcerative colitis. It is also helpful in typhoid fever. Curcumin is helpful to treat diarrhea and chronic dysentery, acidity.

Home Remedy for Dysentry:

50 gm Yogurt mixed with small amount of honey 3 times a day gives fast relief. Herbal decoction is prepared with two tablespoons of dried out **turmeric**, and taken with pure water or buttermilk, the intestinal inside layer is soothed, and the amount of mucus in the stools declines. The use of pomegranate rind is an added effectual preparation for dysentery. About 60 grams of the rind should be boiled in the 250ml of milk. Apple is also considered advantageous in the management of acute and chronic dysentery in the kids. Make a paste of curry leaves and black cumin seeds; consume this paste with a glass of boiled water. The following herbs, supplements, and dietary recommendations may also be a part of your treatment plan; Garlic, Goldenseal, Black Walnut, Wormwood, Pumpkin Seed,

One teaspoon of turmeric and sugar candy 3 times a day is an effective remedy to cure dysentery.

CURCUMIN AND EYE CATARACT

Conjunctivitis refers to an inflammation of the thin transparent membrane covering the front of the eye. This is also referred to as having 'sore eyes' and is a very common form of eye trouble. It spreads from person to person through direct Contact. Overcrowding, dirty surroundings and unhealthy living conditions can cause epidemics of this ailment. Conjunctivitis results from bacterial or a virus infection or eyestrain. Prolonged work under artificial light and excessive use of the eyes in one way or the other, no doubt, contribute towards the disease.

The eyeball and underside of the eyelids become inflamed. At first, the eyes are red and itchy. Later, there may be a watery secretion.

For Cataract: Mix 50 Gums of Anise, Curcumin and Jaggery each. Take 12 grams of this mixture thrice daily for three months. The symptoms of Cataract are resolved in 3 months.

1. Juice that Heal: Raw juices of certain vegetables, especially carrots and spinach, have been found valuable in conjunctivitis. The combined juices of these two vegetables have proved very effective. The juice of the Indian gooseberry, mixed with honey, is useful in conjunctivitis.

2. Food that Heal: Propolis is useful to solve conjunctivitis problems by the scientific research.

3. Herbs that Heal: Bilberry, Eyebright, Lemon Balm, Chamomile, Wormwood.

4. Herbal Tea that Heals: Vinca Rose tea is recommended.

5. Vitamins that Heal: Vitamins A and B2 have proved useful in conjunctivitis.

6. Bath that washes and Heals: Chamomile extract is a fast healing bath on eyes lids.

CURCUMIN AND FEVER

Ginger coffee: It is a Mixture of dried ginger and coriander seeds to be used as a coffee to promote health without side effects and reactions. Very good for digestion, cold, cough and fever.

Turmeric reduces fever and promote a feeling of coolness.

It also eases allergies and hay fever.

In any type of fever, Turmeric curcumin adds to relief by inducing urination in a natural way. An Indian boiled mixture prepared out of coriander seed, buttermilk, turmeric curcumin, cumin seeds and is included in diet of a patient who is suffering from fever helps in reducing fever and supplying readily available calories to patient who is anorexic due to pyrexia.

If we take turmeric curcumin prepared with coriander decoction, very little milk and sugar. This causes sweating and brings down temperature.

During summer, soak anise seeds, turmeric curcumin and poppy seeds overnight. In the morning, grind the seeds in the same water and filter it to obtain a super coolant drink for the body.

Natural Methods of Treating High Fever:

You can find full details of a natural protocol of treating high fever in our book:

How to Fix High Fever in 5 Minutes without Medications which will be printed in the United States.

We can draw the main guidelines of our protocol as follows:

1. Juice that Heals: Lemon-Mint juice can be very helpful.

2. Foods that Heal: Radish

3.Herbs that Heal: Aloe Vera, Chamomile, Gotu Kola, Lavender and Fenugreek.

4. Herbal Tea that Heals: Hundreds of high fever cases who took the herbal tea ;**Fevo Tech Tea** which is simply composed of Chamomile and Turmeric for 3 days could easily solve their high fever problem without medications!!

5. Cream that Heals: Fevo Cream is an excellent natural remedy for fever when it is used twice daily on forehead and foot.

CURCUMIN AND GOUT

Gout results from consuming rich foods loaded with urine that leads to an excess of uric acid, which can build up in the joints and crystallize, causing attacks of painful gout. The needle-like crystals inflame the body joints and cause severe stiffness, swelling and pain, particularly in the big toe, ankles, and feet. In the past, treatment of gout included severe dietary restrictions. Today, natural foods together with herbs can solve the gout problem.

Gout is known as the "**Disease of Kings**" because it is associated with persons of wealth, rich foods, red meat and excessive alcoholic consumption; gout (a form of arthritis) is identified with a number of well-known names in history. From among these are: King Henry VIII, Nostradamus, Isaac Newton, and Charles V, who ruled one of the largest empires in the world.

In controlling gout, high-protein foods increase the blood level of uric acid, and should be almost totally eliminated from the diet. Avoid purine-rich vegetables such as asparagus, cauliflower, dried beans, lentils, and peas; red meat.

As for drinks, one should avoid alcoholic drinks completely during a gout attack. However, one should drink plenty of fluids.

From the phytochemical composition of turmeric we can notice a number of chemical compounds forming turmeric act as excellent anti-inflammatory agents, which clearly means that turmeric is a good candidate to be safely used for gout!!!.

Turmeric serves both as an herb and a spice. It is a healing herb that is used effectively in different parts of the globe. While Indians use it for its anti-inflammatory properties, many other nations use this perennial herb for gout.

Many stories about using **turmeric** for arthritic gout and high uric acid!!!! Many Qatari and Saudi gout patients; got rid of it within 4 weeks only!!!!After starting taking **curcumin** together with the food supplement **URI TECH**.

Natural Methods of Treating Gout Problems:

You can find full details of a natural protocol of treating gout problems in our book:

How to Get throw Gout Out which will be printed in the United States.

We can draw the main guidelines of the protocol as follows:

1. Juice that Heal: Cranberry and **Celery juice** can be very helpful.

2. Food that Heal: Cherry, Lettuce, Cucumber, Cabbage and Tomato are also helpful. Garlic is useful to lower uric acid by the scientific research. Pomegranate, Ginger, Almonds and Walnuts and Grape Seed Extract, Baking Powder is well known by their effects on improving kidney functions.

3. Herbs that Heal: Eating 1 tsp of alfalfa and black seed every morning for 3 months is good for gout. The Indian herb; Shilajit is one of the best herbs for gout. Dandelion and Tribulus terrestris are also very useful.

4. Milk that Heals: Camel milk (as narrated by Prophet Mohammad (PBUH) offers endless health benefits. One of those is treating gout problems. My patients who took 2 glasses of camel milk daily with the food supplement Uri Tech for 3 months found miracle results for both gout and sex!!!!!

5. Herbal Tea that Heals: Hundreds of gout cases who took the herbal tea ;Uri Tech Tea which is simply composed of celery, alfalfa, parsley, curcumin and coriander seed for 3-6 months could easily solve their gout problem without medications!!!!!

6. Food Supplemnts that Heal: Many patients obtained excellent results by using the food supplement named: Uri Tech together with chlorophyll food supplement.

7. Essential Oils that Heal: A number of patients informed me about excellent results on their gouty toes and knees by using the oil mix of coriander oil, turmeric oil and mustard oil for 3-4 weeks only!!!1

Dr. Mansour

Curcumin and Hair Loss Remedy With Coconut Oil and Lime

Although hair is not essential to life, it is of sufficient cosmetic concern to provoke anxiety in anyone when it starts thinning, falling, or disappearing. To a woman, the sight of a comb or brush covered with lost hair can cause intense mental strain.

Hair is formed in minute pockets in the skin called follicles. An up growth at the base of the follicle, called the papilla, actually produces hair when a special group of cells turn amino acids into keratin, a type of protein of which hair is made. The rate of production of these protein 'building blocks' determines hair growth. The average growth rate is about 1.2 cm per month, growing fastest on women between fifteen to thirty years of age.

The most important cause of loss of hair is inadequate nutrition. Even a partial lack of almost any nutrient may cause hair to fall. Persons lacking in vitamin B6 lose their hair and those deficient in folic acid often become completely bald. But the hair grows normally after the liberal intake of these vitamins. Other important causes of loss of hair are stress such as worry, anxiety, and sudden shock; general debility caused by severe or long standing illnesses like typhoid, syphilis, , chronic cold, influenza, and anemia; an unclean condition of the scalp which weakens the hair roots by blocking the pores with the collected dirt; and heredity.

Capsures" (Resveratrol Curcumin Italian combination) was found to have excellent hair growth promoting effects. This hair growth promoting effect, while not definitively known, is likely due to the release of Substance P.

Capsures, the patented Resveratrol/Curcumin combo from Italy uses 82.4mg of a 95% Extract of Curcumin per capsule, 4 times a day, for a total of 350mg. Super Bio- Curcumin.

CURCUMIN AND HEART HEALTH

Everyone with heart problems needs to keep it under control, but it may be even more important for some groups of people, such as

- People with a family history of early heart disease
- People with high blood pressure
- People with diabetes
- People with obesity
- People with continuous stress
- Males over age 45
- Females over age 55
- Smokers

From the phytochemical composition of turmeric we can notice a number of chemical compounds forming Turmeric act as anti-lipid and anti-cholesterol agents, which clearly means that turmeric is a good candidate to be safely used for heart disorders.

Turmeric serves both as an herb and a spice. It is a healing herb that is used effectively in different parts of the globe. While Indians use it for its anti-inflammatory properties, many other nations use this perennial herb for heart health.

Heart Palpitation treatment using Aniseed and Turmeric Curcumin:

Palpitation of the heart may occur due to a variety of factors, most of which may not be related to the heart itself. Anything which increases the work load of the heart may bring on this condition. Some persons may experience palpitations when lying on the left side, because the heart is nearer the chest wall in that position. Many nervous persons suffer from this condition.

A mixture of powdered aniseed, turmeric, and jaggery can also be used beneficially in the treatment of this condition. Equal quantities of each of these three substances should be powdered. About six grams of this mixed powder should be taken after each meal by the patient suffering from palpitation of the heart!!!!!!!

Palpitation is also treated by using Grapes, Honey, or Guava.

For high cholesterol management it has been shown that Turmeric Curcumin acts as an anti-lipid agent and also helps in the vasodilation of veins!!

Many heart cases used Turmeric Curcumin from kitchen together with the powerful Heart Life food supplement and after 3 months they got excellent results.

Natural Methods of Treating Heart Problems:

You can find full details of a natural protocol of treating heart problems in our book:

How to Fix Your Heart without Medications which will be printed in the United States.

We can draw the main guidelines of our protocol as follows:

1. Juice that Heal: Noni, Tomato, Cucumber, and Celery juice can be helpful.

2. Food that Heal: Dark Chocolate, Banana, Peanut Butter, Lettuce, Cucumber, Sunflower seeds, Yogurt and Tomato are also helpful. Garlic is useful to lower the blood high cholesterol by the scientific research. Pomegranate, Ginger, Almonds and Walnuts and Grape Seed Extract are well known by their effects on improving heart functions.

3. Herbs that Heal: Eating 1 tsp of flax seed and black seed every morning for 3 months is good for heart. They also cure high cholesterol and triglycerides due to obesity, as both seeds have weight reducing properties. The Indian herb; Arjuna, Guggul and Hawthorne are the best herbs for heart.

THE 50 MIRACLE CURES OF CURCUMIN

4. Milk that Heals: Camel milk (as narrated by Prophet Mohammad (PBUH) offers endless health benefits. One of those is treating heart problems. Camel milk is said to be the vasodilator of the Future". My patients who took 2 glasses of camel milk daily with the food supplement: Heart Life for 3 months found miracle results for both heart and sex!!!!!

5. Herbal Tea that Heals: Hundreds of heart cases who took the herbal tea ;Heart & Love Tea which is simply composed of Cinnamon, Fenugreek and Turmeric for 3-6 months could easily improve heart functions .

6. Food Supplemnts that Heal: Many patients obtained excellent results by using the food supplement Heart Life which contains a number of anti-lipid herbs including Turmeric!!

Curcumin may cut heart failure risk: Curcumin, the natural pigment that gives the spice turmeric its yellow color, may protect against heart failure - in mice at least - suggests a new study from Canada.

When the pigment was given to mice with enlarged hearts (hypertrophy), heart function was restored and scar formation reduced, report the researchers in the February edition of the *Journal of Clinical Investigation.*

Lead researcher Peter Liu, scientific director at the Canadian Institutes of Health Research - Institute of Circulatory and Respiratory Health said that curcumin might be a safe and effective means of preventing heart failure in the future, given that it is naturally occurring and readily available at a low cost.

Curcumin has come under the scientific spotlight in recent years, with studies investigating its potential benefits for reducing cholesterol levels, improving cardiovascular health, and fighting cancer.

Some experts recommend however that consumers wishing to make use of curcumin's properties consume it in supplement form rather than eating more curries, which tend to be rather high in fat in their Western form.

The Canadian researchers found that curcumin appeared to work by preventing abnormal unravelling of the chromosome under stress, in addition to preventing excessive abnormal protein production.

"Curcumin's ability to shut off one of the major switches right at the chromosome source where the enlargement and scarring genes are being turned on is impressive," said Liu.

Specifically, the pigment was found to act on p300-histone acetyltransferase (HAT), reportedly the most important HAT in muscle that *"modifies chromatin and associated transcription factors and promotes gene activation,"* wrote the researchers.

The study was funded by the Heart and Stroke Foundation and the Canadian Institutes of Health Research.

CURCUMIN AND HEMORRHOIDS

25% of all adults suffer from hemorrhoids at some time in their lives. Hemorrhoids are dilated, stretched, or swollen veins that appear in or around the rectal opening. There may be blood dots within the veins, and sometimes hemorrhoids protrude out of the rectum. They may itch, tear, bleed, and cause extreme pain. In some cases, blood may be visible on the surface of the stools or on toilet paper. Poor circulation and weakness of the blood vessels contribute to hemorrhoids. Straining during bowel movements can aggravate hemorrhoids or lead to their development. Other contributing factors include allergies, recurrent constipation, lack of exercise, lifting heavy objects, obesity, poor nutrition, and standing or sitting for long periods of time. Pregnant women often get hemorrhoids as a result of the added pressure and weight on their pelvic veins.

You can find full details of a natural protocol of treating hemorrhoids problems in our book

How to Rid Hemorrhoids in 4 Weeks which will be printed in the United States.

We can draw the main guidelines of the protocol as follows:

1. Juice that Heal: Add dry ginger powder in buttermilk and drink it to cure piles-wart. Soak coriander seeds in water at night, in the morning mash it; drink that water or otherwise coriander juice to stop the blood falling from the wart. Blood falling from the wart is stopped by drinking the decoction of coriander seed and sugar. By drinking 1-2 tsp of castor oil along with hot milk relieves pain caused due to piles and also avoids scratches on the anus.

2. Food that Heal: Piles-Wart is cured by eating grinded sesame or curcumin in butter. In the morning when the stomach is empty, take a handful of black sesame, chew it and eat it along with sugar to stop the blood falling from the piles Piles-Wart is cured by taking mango seed powder along with honey, Baking Powder are well known by their effects on improving piles. Cut onions into small pieces and dry it in the sun, take little pieces of onion, fry it in the ghee, add little black sesame and sugar powder and eat it in the morning to cure wart. Figs, apricots are important fruits.

3. Herbs that Heal: Roast black cumin seeds; add equal proportion of black pepper and rock salt in it to make a powder. Intake this powder along with butter milk after meal to cure piles-wart. Grind turmeric, heat it, make a bundle and foment with it to relieve the pain caused due to wart. A wart is cured by in taking finely filtered pure turmeric powder along with water before sleeping at night.

4. Milk that Heals: Camel milk (as narrated by Prophet Mohammad (PBUH) offers endless health benefits. One of those is treating piles. My patients who took 2 glasses of camel milk daily for 4 weeks found miracle results for both piles and sex!!!!!

5. Herbal Tea that Heals: Hundreds of piles cases who took our herbal tea;Diges Tech Tea which is simply composed of Chamomile, Oak Bark, Propolis and curcumin for 3 weeks could easily solve their piles without medications!!!

6. Food Supplemnts that Heal: Many patients obtained excellent results by using the food supplement named: Hemo Tech together with the cream: Hemo Tech Cream. Piles are cured by eating mangos teen ketchup along with milk cream.

7. Bath that Heals: 2 drops cypress oil, 2 drops juniper oil. Add the cypress and juniper oils to a shallow tub filled with warm water. Sit hip-deep in the bath for twenty minutes. Another very successful bath my patients used and it did work for years: Equal parts of Oak Leaf, Oak Fruit Peel, Oak Bark and Chamomile are boiled in water bath for 20 minutes and used by sitting anus on it directly for 10 minutes twice daily for 2 weeks only!!!!!

8. Essential Oils that Heals:

1 ounce jojoba oil 4 drops cypress oil 4 drops tea tree oil
3 drops coriander oil or turmeric oil
3 drops myrrh oil

Place the jojoba oil in a clean container, add the essential oils, and gently turn the container upside down several times or roll it between your hands to blend. Apply the oil externally, as needed.

70 — **Dr. Mansour**

CURCUMIN AND HYPERTENSION

A rise in blood pressure above the normal is referred to as high blood pressure or hypertension. But what is blood pressure?

Blood pressure is determined by the force of the contraction of the heart muscle, the resistance or elasticity of the vessel wall, the quantity of blood being pumped from the heart into the vessels, and lastly the viscosity of the blood. The latter depends upon the cellular or fluid constituents which make up the blood volume.

What are the Causes and Symptoms of Hypertension?

A faulty diet, smoking, negative emotional feelings, anxiety and stress are factors which often have a direct bearing on blood pressure. The elasticity of the blood-vessel walls diminishes with age, and certain deposits accumulate on the inner lining. For some reasons, some people are genetically predisposed to this condition. They have a familial tendency to certain lipid (fat) metabolic disorders.

High blood pressure in the early stages usually goes undetected. It is often an accidental finding during a medical check-up for other reasons. However, headaches, fatigue, nosebleeds, shortness of breath, swelling of the feet, palpitations, and nervousness are symptoms that warrant the necessity of an early blood-pressure check-up. In the early stages the high blood pressure has no symptoms.

From the phytochemical composition of turmeric we can notice a number of chemical compounds forming turmeric act as anti-stress hypotensive vasodilator agents, which clearly means that turmeric is a good candidate to be safely used for hypertension (high blood pressure).

Turmeric serves both as an herb and a spice. It is a healing herb that is used effectively in different parts of the globe. While Indians use it for its anti-inflammatory properties, many other nations use this perennial herb for hypertension.

For hypertension management it has been shown that Curcumin acts as an anti-stress hypotensive agent and also helps in the vasodilation of veins!!

Curcumin Shows Promising Signs In Reducing Hypertension & Heart Enlargement

Eating curcumin may dramatically reduce the chance of developing heart failure, researchers at the Peter Munk Cardiac Center of the Toronto General Hospital have discovered.

In a study entitled, "Curcumin prevents and reverses murine cardiac hypertrophy, "published in the February edition of the Journal of Clinical Investigation, researchers found when the herb is given orally to a variety of mouse models with enlarged hearts (hypertrophy), it can prevent and reverse hypertrophy, restore heart function and reduce scar formation.

Dr. Liu, who holds the Heart and Stroke Foundation's Polo Chair Professor in Medicine and Physiology at the University of Toronto, says that since curcumin is a naturally occurring compound that is readily available at a low cost, it might be a safe and effective means of preventing heart failure in the future. Dr. Robert O. Young, a research scientist at the pH Miracle Living Center, states, "curcumin is a wonderful buffer of metabolic and dietary acids that can lead to hypertension and heart enlargement. The key to eliminating hypertension and heart enlargement is to reduce the levels are endogenous acids with better lifestyle and dietary choices. One of those dietary choices would definitely include the curcumin spice."

Many hypertensive cases used Curcumin from kitchen together with the powerful PRESS OIL which is used externally 5 times a day as a relaxing agent. All cases including myself got rid of high blood pressure for good in less than 24 weeks!!!! I discovered myself with high blood pressure of 190/105 3 years ago and I started taking the relaxation oil (PRESS OIL) together with coriander tea and after 12 weeks only I measured my blood pressure and found it normal!!!!!Now my pressure reads 120/80 and sometimes 110/70 without any medications!!!!!

THE 50 MIRACLE CURES OF CURCUMIN

Natural Methods of Treating Hypertension:

You can find full details of a natural protocol of treating hypertension in our book:

How to Lower Your High Blood Pressure to Normal in 12 weeks which will be printed in the United States.

We can draw the main guidelines of the protocol as follows:

1. Juice that Heal: Noni, Tomato, Cucumber, and Celery juice can be helpful.

2. Food that Heal: Banana and Potato (rich in potassium), Cocoa, Dark Chocolate, Brown Algae, Lettuce, Cucumber, Yogurt and Tomato are also helpful... Garlic is useful to lower the blood pressure by the scientific research.

3. Herbs that Heal: Eating 1 tsp of khella seed and flax seed every morning for 3 months is said to prevent hypertension due to heredity factors. They also cure hypertension due to obesity, as both seeds have weight reducing properties.

4. Milk that Heals: Camel milk (as narrated by Prophet Mohammad (PBUH) offers endless health benefits. One of those is treating hypertension. Camel milk is said to be the vasodilator of the Future". My patients who took 2 glasses of camel milk daily or the food supplement: Camel Tech for 3 months found miracle results for both hypertension and sex!!!!!

5. Herbal Tea that Heals: Hundreds of hypertensives who took the herbal tea ;Relax U Tea which is simply composed of Hibiscus, Olive Leaf, Linden, curcumin and coriander seed for 3-6 months could easily reduce their high blood pressure to normal without medications!!!!!

6. Food Supplemnts that Heal: Many patients obtained excellent results by using the food supplement named: Press Tech which contains a number of hypotensive herbs including Curcumin and Coriander seed!!!!

7. Essential Oils that Heal: The oil mix; Press Oil was successfully used with hundreds of hypertensive patients together with coriander tea and all of them became hypertension free!!!!!!

8. Sex that Heals: It was found by a number of researchers that performing sex 3 times weekly reduces and may cure blood pressure permanently!!!!!

9. Water that Heals: Honey Water

It is narrated in QURAN that honey is a complete cure!!! I supervised a graduate student who tested using water and different percentages of honey in capillary tubes similar to veins and we published our findings in the International J.Biomedical Engineering 14 years ago!!!! The results of study showed that a drinking honey water: a mixture of 1 tbs of honey in a glass of water reduces blood pressure, cholesterol and maintains vasodilatation.!!!!!!!!!

10.Vitamin that Heals:

There is a direct relation between lack of Magnesium and high blood pressure. Dr.Whitaker describes 1000mg of Magnesium combined with Potassium.

Pulmonary Hypertension:

Pulmonary hypertension is a very difficult condition everywhere in the world and it is well known that nobody arrived at a cure!!!!! By using the natural protocol for hypertension a number of severe cases; one of them is a medical doctor solved his pulmonary hypertension for

CURCUMIN AND INSOMNIA

Insomnia is a sleeping disorder characterized by persistent difficulty falling asleep or staying asleep despite the opportunity. It is typically followed by functional impairment while awake. Insomniacs have been known to complain about being unable to close their eyes or "rest their mind" for more than a few minutes at a time. Both organic and non-organic insomnia constitute a sleep disorder

For Sleep Disorder (Insomnia): Paste of turmeric should be applied on forehead to induce sleep or else, take orally fresh juice of leaves with some sugar-candy.

Turmeric curcumin has been used as a folk medicine for the relief of anxiety and insomnia in folk medicine. Experiments in mice support its use as an anxiolytic.

Insomnia Home Remedy Using Gotu Kola, Coriander, Curcumin, Cumin and Water Spinach:

How to use it:

Take 1 spoon of cumin seeds, 3 stalks of water spinach, 2 pegagan leaves, and 1/4 tsp coriander. Boil the whole ingredients with 2 glass of water until there is only 1 glass left of it. Then put it through a sieve and drink it before sleep. Do it every day until the desired results are achieved.

Natural Methods of Treating Insomnia:

You can find full details of a natural protocol of treating insomnia in our book:

Solve Your Insomnia in 4 Weeks without Medications which will be printed in the United States.

We can draw the main guidelines of our protocol as follows:

1. **Juice that Heal:** Lemon-Lemon Balm juice can be very helpful.
2. **Foods that Heal**: Whole Lemon
3. **Herbs that Heal:** Hops, Chamomile, Lemon Balm, Valerian and Passion Flower.
4. **Herbal Tea that Heals:** Hundreds of insomnia cases who took the herbal tea ;**Relax U Tea** which is simply composed of Lemon Balm, Chamomile and Curcumin for 3 weeks could easily solve their insomnia without medications!!
5. Oils that Heal: Relax U oil is one of the best natural essential oils that helps in cases of insomnia.

CURCUMIN AND IRRITABLE COLON

(*IRRITABLE BOWEL SYNDROME –IBS*)

Curcumin is considered a carminative that will help prevent gas from forming in the intestines and will also help expel wind from the bowels. In addition, curcumin is believed to allay the "griping" (pain and grumbling in the bowels) often associated with other laxatives.

As an antispasmodic, curcumin is thought to help relieve diarrhea and ease abdominal cramps.

Turmeric contains substances that are anti-bacterial, anti-inflammatory and antifungal, helping to prevent infections from developing in wounds. Topically applied, the essential oil of Turmeric has been used to ease the pain of rheumatic joints, sore muscles, neuralgia and sciatica, which appear to attest to its anti-inflammatory reputation.

COLON AND GASES:

Cure a cranky irritable digestion this way:
Stress hits women in the digestive tract. During high-stress times reach for these herbs and spices:
Curcumin tones up your digestion.
Curcumin eases gas.
Cardamom reduces mucous-forming effects of dairy foods.
Turmeric helps your liver work more efficiently.
Black pepper helps you digest dairy foods.
Fennel prevents gas.
Curcumin serves both as an herb and a spice. It is a healing herb that is used effectively in different parts of the globe. While Indians

use it for its anti-inflammatory properties, many other nations use this herb for digestion.

We have many successful stories about using curcumin for irritable colon!!

Natural Methods of Treating Irritable Colon:

You can find full details of our natural protocol of treating irritable colon problems in our book:

The Only Fast Solution for Irritable Colon in the World which will be printed in the United States.

We can draw the main guidelines of our protocol as follows:

1. Juice that Heal: Wheatgrass, Mint-Lemon juice can be very helpful.

2. Food that Heal: Propolis and Licorice are useful to solve irritable colon problems by the scientific research.

3. Herbs that Heal: Eating 1 tsp of Caraway, Fennel, and Anise every morning for 3 months is good for irritable colon.

4. Milk that Heals: Camel milk (as narrated by Prophet Mohammad (PBUH) offers endless health benefits. One of those is treating irritable colon. My patients who took 2 glasses of camel milk daily for 3 months found miracle results for both irritable colon and sex!!!!!

5. Herbal Tea that Heals: Hundreds of irritable colon cases who took the herbal tea; Diges Tech Tea which is simply composed of Mint, Fennel, Anise, and, curcumin and coriander seed for 3 months could easily solve their irritable colon problem without medications!!!!!

CURCUMIN AND JAUNDICE

Jaundice is a condition characterized by the yellowing of the whites of the eyes, the mucous membranes, urine and the skin. It is often caused by dysfunction of the liver. The yellow coloring comes from bilirubin, which is caused by aging red blood cells. The accumulation of excessive red blood cells within the body results in jaundice.

As for drinks, one should avoid alcoholic drinks completely.

From the phytochemical composition of turmeric we can notice a number of chemical compounds forming turmeric act as excellent an anti-inflammatory agent, which clearly means that turmeric is a good candidate to be safely used for jaundice!!!.

Turmeric also can help cure jaundice by reducing yellowness of the skin and whites of the eyes.

Natural Methods of Treating Jaundice Problems:

You can find full details of a natural protocol of treating jaundice problems in our book:

How to Rid Jaundice in 3 Days without Medications which will be printed in the United States.

We can draw the main guidelines of our protocol as follows:

1. Juice that Heal: Lemon Juice, One glass of sugar cane juice, mixed with the juice of half a lime, and taken twice daily, can hasten recovery from jaundice and Tomato juice and Barley water drink can be very helpful.

2. Food that Heal: Honey, Lemon, Cucumber, Cabbage and Tomato are also helpful... Pomegranate, Almonds, Dried Dates and Cardamoms, Baking Powder are well known by their effects on jaundice. The green leaves of radish are another valuable remedy for jaundice

3. Herbs that Heal: Eating 1 tsp of cinnamon and black seed with honey every morning for 2 weeks is good for jaundice. The Indian herb; Shilajit is one of the best herbs for jaundice. Milk Thistle, Dandelion and Andrographis are also very useful.

4. Milk that Heals: Camel milk (as narrated by Prophet Mohammad (PBUH) offers endless health benefits. One of those is treating jaundice problems. My patients who took 2 glasses of camel milk daily or our food supplement LivTech for 2 weeks found miracle results for both jaundice and sex!!!!!

5. Herbal Tea that Heals: Hundreds of jaundice cases who took the herbal tea ;Liv Tea which is simply composed of Radish Leaf, Lemon Balm and turmeric for 2 weeks could easily solve their jaundice problem.

6. Food Supplemnts that Heal: Many patients obtained excellent results by using the food supplement named: Liv Tech which contains a number of anti-inflammatory herbs including turmeric!! together with chlorophyll supplement.

7. Avoid: Smoking and drinking Alcohol.

CURCUMIN AND KIDNEY HEALTH

In renal failure the kidneys undergo cellular death and are unable to filter wastes, produce urine and maintain fluid balances. This dysfunction causes a buildup of toxins in the body which can affect the blood, brain and heart, as well as other complications. Renal failure is very serious and even deadly if left untreated.

The symptoms of renal failure include edema, which is an accumulation of fluid characterized by swelling, and a decrease in urination. Other symptoms may include a general ill feeling, exhaustion and headaches. Often, a person with renal failure does not experience any symptoms

From the phytochemical composition of turmeric we can notice a number of chemical compounds forming turmeric act as excellent anti-inflammatory agents, which clearly means that turmeric is a good candidate to be safely used for renal(kidney)failure!!!.

Curcumin curry's secret agent: behind all great spices are powerful healing compounds. For the curry seasoning turmeric, that hidden gem is curcumin—a potent antioxidant that quells inflammation and keeps the mind sharp

Natural Methods of Treating Kidney Problems:

You can find full details of a natural protocol of treating kidney problems in our book:

How to Avoid Dialysis without Medications which will be printed in the United States.

We can draw the main guidelines of a protocol as follows:

1. Juice that Heal: Noni, Tomato, **Cranberry**, Aloe Vera and Celery juice can be helpful.

2. Food that Heal: Asparagus Soup, Lettuce, Cucumber, Cabbage and Tomato are also helpful. Garlic is useful to lower the blood pressure and improve kidney function by the scientific research. Pomegranate, Ginger, Almonds and Walnuts and Grape Seed Extract, Baking Powder is well known by their effects on improving kidney functions.

3. Herbs that Heal: Eating 1 tsp of flax seed and black seed every morning for 3 months is good for kidney. The Indian herb; Shilajit is one of the best herbs for kidney. Dandelion and Tribulus terrestris are also very useful.

4. Milk that Heals: Camel milk (as narrated by Prophet Mohammad (PBUH) offers endless health benefits. One of those is treating kidney problems. My patients who took 2 glasses of camel milk daily or the food supplement Reno Tech for 3 months found miracle results for both kidney and sex!!!!!

5. Herbal Tea that Heals: Hundreds of kidney cases who took the herbal tea ;Reno Tea which is simply composed of Celery, Linden and Curcumin for 3-6 months could easily improve kidney functions!!!!!

6. Food Supplemnts that Heal: Many patients obtained excellent results by using the food supplement named: Reno Tech which contains a number of together with chlorophyll supplement.

CURCUMIN AND LIVER CIRRHOSIS

Cirrhosis is a complication of many liver diseases that is characterized by abnormal structure and function of the liver. The diseases that lead to cirrhosis do so because they injure and kill liver cells and the inflammation and repair that is associated with the dying liver cells causes scar tissue to form. The liver cells that do not die multiply in an attempt to replace the cells that have died. This results in clusters of newly-formed liver cells (regenerative nodules) within the scar tissue. There are many causes of cirrhosis; they include chemicals (such as alcohol, Qat consumption(in Yemen), fat, and certain medications), viruses, toxic metals (such as iron and copper that accumulate in the liver as a result of genetic diseases), and autoimmune liver disease in which the body's immune system attacks the liver.

Enlarged Liver:

The liver is one of the largest organs in the body. Its functions include filtering the blood, producing bile and amino acids, and serving as a storage site for glucose. When the liver becomes enlarged or "fatty," the body can suffer serious side effects, some of which can be fatal if left untreated. Here are some of the factors that cause hepatomegaly, or enlargement of the liver:

Congestive Heart Failure, Alcohol, Hemochromatosis which is a condition wherein there is an excessive amount of iron in the body, Cancer, Hepatitis, Nonalcoholic fatty liver disease, seen in people with obesity, diabetes or high cholesterol, causes an accumulation of fat in the liver. The result is inflammation and subsequent enlargement of the liver.

People with liver problems should not take alcohol at all. A healthy diet with fruits and vegetables is advised.

Curcumin can help fortifying the liver. You will need 1.5 teaspoons of curcumin. Add a cup of boiling water. Repeat it 3 times daily.

You can take the food supplements: Liv Tech and Liv52.

Natural Methods of Treating Liver Problems:

You can find full details of a natural protocol of treating liver problems in our book: **How to Fix Your Liver without Medications** which will be printed in the United States.

We can draw the main guidelines of our protocol as follows:

1. Juice that Heal: White Radish, Wheatgrass, Cucumber, and Celery juice can be helpful.

2. Food that Heal:, Lettuce, Cucumber, Yogurt and Tomato are also helpful. Pomegranate, Ginger, Almonds and Grape Seed Extract are well known by their effects on improving liver functions.

3. Herbs that Heal: Eating 1 tsp of curcumin and black seed with honey every morning for 3 months is good for liver.

4. Milk that Heals: Camel milk mixed with camel urine (as narrated by Prophet Mohammad (PBUH) offers endless health benefits. One of those is treating liver problems: Cirrhosis, Enlargement, Hepatitis B & C ad Liver Cancer. Camel milk is said to be the Liver Cure of the Future". My patients who took 2 glasses of camel milk (mixed with camel urine) daily or the food supplement: Camel Tech for 3-6 months found miracle results for both liver and sex!!!!!

5. Herbal Tea that Heals: Hundreds of liver cases who took our herbal tea ;Liv & Love Tea which is simply composed of Cinnamon, Fenugreek, curcumin and Coriander seed for 3-6 months could easily improve liver functions!!!

THE 50 MIRACLE CURES OF CURCUMIN

6. **Food Supplemnts that Heal:** Many patients obtained excellent results by using our food supplement named: Camel Tech which contains a number of anti-cirrhotic herbs including curcumin together with chlorophyll food supplement.

A recent experiment from the Biology Department at the University of King Abdul Aziz in Saudi, on rats showed excellent results on immune system and cancer.

Liver Detox Secret! Turmeric and Coriander Heal Liver!

It is well known that liver represents the filter and port that receives all toxins from other parts of the body and when it is overloaded by toxins of food, drugs or chemotherapy sources it does need a process of detoxification by certain types of herbs; one of them is curcumin.

For example the following procedure is given by one of the experts asked about the detox process after chemotherapy and this process can be followed by any person at many stations in his life:

By Nancy Lonsdorf, MD:

Q. Over the past few years, I've had surgery and chemo for cancer. How can I restore my immune and hormonal systems?

A. Although most of the effects of chemotherapy are short-term, some—including fatigue, impaired immunity, hormonal imbalances, and temporary problems with memory, attention, and concentration (recently dubbed "chemobrain")—can persist for years. To date, not many researchers have looked at the efficacy of treatments to reverse or prevent these long-term side effects. However, it makes sense that approaches that support detoxification reduce stress, and rebuild immunity will help speed your recovery from both the cancer and its treatment.

Reducing damage to the body during treatment also may prevent side effects down the line. In laboratory studies, researchers found that one traditional Ayurvedic herbal formula called amrit nectar protects normal cells from chemotherapy injury. In another small clinical trial, the formula reduced side effects and improved overall strength and well-being without interfering with chemo's anti-cancer effects. Our clinical experience with traditional detoxification approaches from ayurveda, the traditional health system of India, has convinced me that cleansing the body of toxins and rebalancing the body after cancer treatment can help restore optimum health. This type of ayurvedic detox has two phases. Phase I: During the first eight weeks when your body is recovering strength and stamina, eat a wholesome diet with immune-boosting herbs and spices, drink plenty of pure water, reduce stress, and get extra sleep to enhance your body's own healing response.

Follow the tips below for optimal detox and recovery during this time.

• Eat organically grown foods, including whole grains, legumes, unprocessed nuts and seeds, and seven to 10 servings of fresh vegetables, fruits, and freshly squeezed juices each day.

• Avoid alcohol, refined sugar, artificial ingredients, cigarette smoke, chemicals, and pollution.

• Cook with turmeric, coriander, cilantro, basil, oregano, rosemary, ginger, garlic, cinnamon, fennel, clove, and saffron to support immunity, hormonal balance, detoxification, and antioxidant protection.

• Take soluble fiber such as psyllium husks to promote elimination of toxins excreted by the liver via the stool.
• Drink eight glasses of warm, pure spring water daily.
• Lower your stress with effective techniques such as yoga and meditation. Research has shown that Transcendental Meditation enhances quality of life in breast cancer patients, reduces stress hormone levels, promotes longevity, and boosts DNA repair.

- Support liver detox and the production of glutathione, the body's primary defense against most toxins, with plenty of protein in your diet. No vegetarians are advised to favor more easily digestible sources such as organic poultry and wild-caught fish that are low in mercury. Vegetarians may wish to include organic, high-protein vegetable sources such as soaked nuts and seeds, legumes, quinoa, amaranth, spirulina, and hemp-seed nut. Consult your doctor before increasing soy in your diet.

- Drink this simple detox tea to support liver and kidney function: Add 1/4 teaspoon whole cumin seed, 1/2 teaspoon whole coriander, and 1/4 teaspoon whole fennel to two quarts of boiled hot, pure spring water; let steep, and sip throughout the day for two months.

Phase II: After two months, if you still feel in need of detox, consider the intensive level of Ayurvedic detox called panchakarma, traditionally done in-residence under professional supervision.

Check out The Raj (www.theraj.com), a health spa offering holistic and natural maharishi ayurveda treatments and massage. Panchakarma includes warm oil massages, gentle heat treatments, and mild elimination therapies to remove both water- and fat-soluble toxins from deep in the tissues. (Other non-Ayurvedic detoxification approaches, such as steam baths, saunas, aerobic exercise, and drinking large amounts of water, can also reduce water-soluble toxins substantially.) In one two-month study, five days of panchakarma treatments resulted in a 46 percent drop in blood levels of PCBs and 58 percent drop in beta-HCH, prevalent environmental toxins linked to cancer and other serious disorders. It is always best to detox under professional supervision with methods supported by research and an established safety track record.

CURCUMIN AND LOST APPETITE

A sign of good health is the presence of a healthy appetite-a good appetite will be neither over powering nor very mild in the way it affects the person. The fact is that even the slightest physical or emotional problems can affect the appetite of a person, and for this reason the presence of a poor appetite may not necessarily be a major health concern. Appetite problems can come in different ways and some other physical symptoms of a malfunctioning appetite include the presence of abdominal bloating, persistent indigestion and constipation - sensations of nausea or pain can also be felt if the appetite is affected in some cases. The cause of the drop in appetite will brook further investigation when the sudden or gradual appetite loss comes along with any kind of weight loss - a medical examination becomes important in such cases as it could be a signal for the presence of some other serious disorder - a poor appetite can then be a symptom for an underlying condition.

Curcumin is a great spicy remedy for restoring lost appetite since it is rich in polyphenols and anti-oxidants.

1. Juice that Heal: Wheatgrass, Mint-Lemon juice can be very helpful.

2. Food that Heal: Okra is also helpful. Propolis and Licorice are useful to solve digestion problems by the scientific research.

3. Herbs that Heal: Alfalfa, Lemon Balm, Mint, Ginger, Cardamom, Wormwood.

4. Milk that Heals: Camel milk (as narrated by Prophet Mohammad (PBUH) offers endless health benefits. One of those is treating Appetite problems. My patients who took 2 glasses of camel milk daily for 3 weeks found miracle results for both Appetite and sex!!!!!

5. Herbal Tea that Heals: Many cases who took the herbal tea; Diges Tech Tea which is simply composed of Mint, Ginger, Lemon Balm and curcumin for 3 weeks could easily solve their Appetite problem!!

6. Vitamins that Heal-Vitamin B-Complex, Folic Acid, Zinc.

7. Essential Oils that Heal: Commonly used essential oils for appetite loss are: Bergamot, Caraway, Chamomile, Cinnamon, Coriander, Ginger, Hyssop, Ylang Ylang.

CURCUMIN, MEMORY & ALZHEIMER

It is well known that curcumin improves blood circulation throughout the body and hence improves memory.

A number of students used curcumin together with black seed, gotu kola and ginkgo biloba as an herbal tea and all of them showed improvement in memory, vitality and clear way of thinking!!!

They also used curcumin oil mixed with brahmi oil, rosemary oil and ginger oil on their foreheads and all of them showed an excellent progress in their school!!!

The tea mentioned above was used as a fruit drink mixed with cranberry/strawberry juices and the results were the same.

Other good home remedies to improve memory are:

Milk and honey have been shown to help improve your memory. While there are many books you can buy which will present a number of techniques you can use to improve your memory.

Also Almond and almond milk. Fish oil, Walnut, Rosemary, Ginseng, Thyme and Pistachio are very useful for memory.

FROM: Curr Alzheimer Res. 2005 Apr;2(2):131-6 A Study showed:

A potential role of the curry spice curcumin in Alzheimer's disease.

University of California, Los Angeles, Department of Neurology, Alzheimer's Disease Research Center, Los Angeles, CA 90095, USA.

There is substantial in-vitro data indicating that curcumin has antioxidant, anti-inflammatory, and anti-amyloid activity. In addition, studies in animal models of Alzheimer's disease (AD) indicate a direct effect of curcumin in decreasing the amyloid pathology of AD. As the widespread use of curcumin as a food additive and relatively small short-term studies in humans suggest safety, curcumin is a promising agent in the treatment and/or prevention of AD. Nonetheless, important information regarding curcumin bioavailability, safety and tolerability, particularly in an elderly population is lacking. We are therefore performing a study of curcumin in patients with AD to gather this information in addition to data on the effect of curcumin on biomarkers of AD pathology.

The early research findings, which appear in the July issue of the *Journal of Alzheimer's Disease*, may lead to new approaches in preventing and treating Alzheimer's by utilizing the property of vitamin D3 both alone and together with curcumin to boost the immune system in protecting the brain against amyloid beta.

CURCUMIN AND MENSTRUAL FLOW PROBLEMS

Heavy menstrual bleeding and clotting are common problems for many women. When a woman soaks a pad or a tampon an hour for several hours or more or bleeds for more than a week and a half each month, this is called *menorrhagia*. If she soaks through two or more pads or tampons an hour, this is generally considered *hypermenorrhagia*

Curcumin check excessive menstrual flow. 6 grams of the spice should be boiled in half a liter of water, till only half the water remains. Sugar or honey should be added to it and taken when it is still warm. The patient gets relief after taking this for 3 or 4 days.

Moreover in recent studies curcumin was showed very effective against ovarian and uterus cancers.

Other Home Remedies for Menstruation:

Menstruation treatment with Parsley: Parsley is one of the most efficient among the several home remedies in the treatment of menstrual disorders. It increases menstruation and helps in the regularization of the monthly periods.

Menstruation treatment with Ginger: The use of ginger is a useful home remedy for menstrual disorders, especially in cases of painful menstruation and stoppage of menstrual flow.

Menstruation treatment with Sesame Seeds: Sesame seeds are precious in Menstruation. Half a teaspoon of powder of these seeds, taken with hot water two times daily, acts brilliantly in reducing spasmodic pain during menstruation in young, unmarried anemic girls.

Menstruation treatment via Papaya: The unripe papaya helps the contractions of the muscle fibers of the uterus and is thus helpful in securing a proper menstrual flow. Papaya is especially useful when menstruation ceases due to stress or fright in young unmarried girls.

Menstruation treatment with Marigold: The herb Marigold, named after the Virgin Mary, is helpful in allaying any pain during menstruation and smoothes the progress of menstrual flow. An infusion of the herb must be given in doses of one tablespoon two times every day for the treatment of these disorders.

Menstruation treatment with Banana Flower: The use of banana flower is one of the most efficient home remedies in the treatment of menorrhagia or excessive menstruation. One banana flower should be cooked and consumed with one cup of curd. This will increase the quantity of progesterone and decrease the bleeding.

Menstruation treatment with Mango Bark: The juice of the fresh mango bark is one more valuable remedy for heavy bleeding during menstruation. The juice is given with the addition of white of an egg as an option, a mixture of 10 ml of a fluid extract of the bark, and 120 ml of water may be given in doses of one teaspoon every hour or two.

Menstruation treatment with Barberry: The herb Indian barberry is helpful in case of excessive bleeding. It should be given in doses of 13-25 grams every day.

Menstruation treatment with Hermal: Hermal is useful in regulating the menstrual periods. It is particularly beneficial in painful and difficult menstruation. Two tablespoons of the seeds should be boiled in half a liter of water, till it is decreased by one-third. This decoction should be prearranged in 15 to 30 ml doses.

CURCUMIN AND MOUTH ULCER

Mouth ulcer is the loss of delicate tissue that lines inside the mouth caused by a break in the mucous membrane or epithelium on the lips.

What Causes Mouth Ulcers?

Among the factors causing mouth ulcer are stress, fatigue, illness, injury from accidental biting, hormonal changes, burns from eating hot food, poor oral hygiene, menstruation, sudden weight loss, food allergies, deficiencies in vitamin B12, iron and folic acid, certain drugs, chemicals. In some cases, mouth ulcers are not harmful and resolve by themselves in a few days without any treatment.

- Infection with a type of bacteria called Helicobacter Pylori **(H. pylori)** also causes mouth ulcer.

- Use of painkillers called non-steroidal anti-inflammatory drugs (NSAIDs), and many others available by prescription. Even aspirin coated with a special substance can still cause ulcers and that is why it is used coated.

- Excess acid production from gastronomes, tumors of the acid producing cells of the stomach that increases acid output.

Curcumin helps cure mouth ulcer, inflammation and spasm.

Diet for Mouth Ulcers

Whenever mouth ulcers occur avoid hot, spicy food, caffeine and tea. Consume green vegetables as much as possible as green vegetables provide the necessary fiber for the movement of bowels which prevents constipation, advisable to stop fatty food. Papaya is a very good fruit to be consumed in mouth ulcers. It soothes the mouth ulcers and helps in quick recovery.

Home Cure:

Paste of garlic in coconut milk is useful in mouth ulcer, chew holy basil leaf, apply milk of raw papaya on ulcer, gargle with curcumin boil water, paste of Indian plum leaves.

As for drinks, one should avoid alcoholic drinks completely during mouth ulcer attack.

Curcumin serves both as an herb and a spice. It is a healing herb that is used effectively in different parts of the globe. While Indians use it for its anti-inflammatory properties, many other nations use this perennial herb for mouth ulcer.

Natural Methods of Treating Mouth Ulcer:

You can find full details of a natural protocol of treating gout problems in our book: **How to Fix Mouth Ulcer without Medications** which will be printed in the United States.

We can draw the main guidelines of our protocol as follows:

1. Juice that Heal: Licorice, Cabbage juice can be very helpful.

2. Food that Heal: Cherry, Lettuce, Cucumber, Cabbage are also helpful. Pomegranate, Ginger, Almonds, Walnuts, Baking Powder are well known by their effects on improving mouth ulcer.

3. Herbs that Heal: Eating 1 tsp of Fenugreek, Aloe Vera, Ginger, Lemon Balm, Chamomile, Peppermint, Licorice and black seed every morning for 3 weeks is good for mouth ulcer. The Indian herb; Shilajit is one of the best herbs for mouth ulcer. Propolis is an excellent choice for mouth ulcer.

4. Milk that Heals: Camel milk (as narrated by Prophet Mohammad (PBUH) offers endless health benefits. One of those is treating mouth ulcer. My patients who took 2 glasses of camel milk daily for 3 months found miracle results for both mouth ulcer and sex!!!!!

5. Herbal Tea that Heals: Hundreds of mouth ulcer cases who took the herbal tea ;Diges Tech Tea which is simply composed of

Licorice, Alfalfa, Pomegranate Peels, Propolis and Curcumin for 3 weeks could easily solve their mouth ulcer problem!!!!!

6. **Food Supplements that Heal:** Many patients obtained excellent results by using the food supplement named: Stomach Care which contains a number of herbs including Curcumin!!!! Together with chlorophyll supplement.

7. **Essential Oils that Heal:** Some components of essential oils in Curcumin, is an excellent antiseptic. In addition, other components have anti microbial and healing effects which do not let wounds and ulcers in the mouth go worse. They aid healing up of ulcers and freshen up the breath.

Dr. Mansour

CURCUMIN AND MULTIPLE SCLEROSIS

What is it MS? MS is a degenerative and progessive autoimmune disease of the central nervous system that destroys the myelin seaths which cover the nerves, causing an inflammatory response and paralysis.A strong immune system helps avoid infection and a special diet rich in vitamins and minerals is beneficial for the MS patients. OR in more details:

MS is a degenerative disease that affects the brain, optic nerve and spinal cord. The disease destroys myelin sheaths that cover the nerves, ultimately destroying the nerves. Symptoms vary and progress with time. In the beginning there may be dizziness, mood swings, blurred vision, numbness, nausea and vomiting. Later a person may have trouble walking; eventually paralysis and difficulty breathing may occur. Usually the disease presents itself in flare-ups, which may occur every few months or every few years. The exact cause of MS is unknown. Many believe, however, that stress, malnutrition or a virus could be factors. Others suggest that chemical or mercury poisoning could be major factors.

At this time there is no cure for this disease.
Many stories successfully used turmeric curcumin as an anti-inflammatory agent together with the food supplements M.S., Rheuma Tech and Joint Tech!!!!!

Natural Methods of Treating MS Problems

You can find full details of a natural protocol of treating MS problems in our book: **How to Deal with MS without Medications** which will be printed in the United States .

We can draw the main guidelines of our protocol as follows:

1. Juice that Heal: Cranberry and celery juice can be very helpful.

2. Food that Heal: Pomegranate, Ginger, and Grape Seed Extract, Baking Powder is well known by their effects on reducing arthritis and joint pain. Apples, apricots, cherries, grapes, citrus fruits, cheese, beets, blurberry, broccoli, green leafy vegetables, Soy Beans, Licorice Root, spinach, red meat, mushrooms, flax seed oil, Evening primrose oil and garlic.

3. Herbs that Heal: Eating 1 tsp of alfalfa seed, curcumin and ginger with honey every morning for 3 months is good for MS. The Indian herb; Shilajit is one of the best herbs for MS. Evening Primrose Oil, Kelp, Olive Leaf, Burdock Root, Dandelion Oat, Curcumin, and St.John's, Rice Bran, Pine Bark Extract, Olive Leaf, Cod Liver Oil, Ginseng, Burdock Root, Dandelion, Royal Jelly, Propolis, are important too.

4. Milk that Heals: Camel milk (as narrated by Prophet Mohammad (PBUH) offers endless health benefits. One of those is treating MS problems. My patients who took 2 glasses of camel milk daily for 6-12 months found miracle results for both MS and sex!!!!!

5. Herbal Tea that Heals: Many MS cases who took the herbal tea ;Energy Tea which is simply composed of Celery, Alfalfa, Parsley, **Curcumin** and Coriander seed for 3-6 months could easily solve their MS symptoms without medications! Ephedra Tea is essential.

6. Food Supplemnts that Heal: Many patients obtained excellent results by using the food supplements named: M.S., Rheuma Tech and Joint Tech. All of them contain anti-inflammatory herbs including Curcumin, EPA, CQ10, Histamin, Lecithin, L Valine, Pregenolone, Glutathione, Alpha Liopic Acid, Carnitine.

7. Essential Oils that Heal: A number of patients informed me about excellent results on their joints, back and knees by using the

THE 50 MIRACLE CURES OF CURCUMIN

oils: Relax U, Massage oil, Jojoba oil and Press oil for 6 weeks only!!! Relax U is for pain and numbness, Other oils are for pain, fatigue, stress, depression, swelling and they stimulate blood circulation, ease muscular stiffness & weakness, relieve arthritis and inflammatory conditions.Sage oil has a special effect on MS if it is taken orally; 2-3 drops twice daily.

8.Creams that Heal: IRIS Massage, MG, Bee Venom creams

9.Drinks that Heal: Our Energy Zero Calorie Drink.

10.Baths that Heal: Dead sea salt bath for 20 minutes once daily and Baking Soda bath once daily.

11.Vitamins that Heal: Vitamin D3, B6

AVOID: *Wine, Smoking, Carbonated Beverages, Saturated Fats, Processed Food. All Diet foods and drinks(aspartame).*

CURCUMIN AND NOSE BLEED

Nose Bleed is a common condition which one sees especially in children. Nose Bleed is also known as Epistaxis and Bleeding from the nose. The blood vessels in the nasal passage are very tender and easily rupture with the slightest pressure or injury. Since the veins of the nose are devoid of valves therefore the bleeding is usually very heavy. Curcumin is very beneficial in resolving the incidence of Nose Bleed when mixed with Amla or Arjuna herbs.

As one of the home remedies for nosebleed, you can add a piece of camphor in small amounts of coriander leaves.

Here are some of the Common Home Remedies for the Treatment of Nose Bleeding:

Coriander Leaves - Use juice of fresh coriander leaves as nasal drops.

Alum - Herbalists suggest using wild alum root powder. This will stop the bleeding immediately. Wild alum root is a powerful astringent.

Lemon Juice - Mix the juice of three lemons into two cups of cold water and sponge on the sunburn. The lemon will cool the burn, act as a disinfectant, and will promote healing of the skin.

Goldenseal - This one is another good remedy used for curing nose bleeds. Make a tea from goldenseal using one teaspoon to a pint of boiling water. Steep a few minutes and let it settle at the bottom, and when it is cooled down - snuff some into your nostrils. Do this several times during the day to prevent recurrence.

Tulsi Juice - Drinking tulsi juice mixed with honey will also help and provide extra strength to the body.

Vinegar - Pour some vinegar on a cloth and wash the neck, nose and temples with it.

Pomegranate Juice: To stop or prevent nosebleeds, you can drink cranberry juice, pomegranate juice, or a half-and-half mixture of the two.

SNIFF COLD WATER: Take a little cool water in your palm, inhale it up into the nose, and gently blow the nose.

CURCUMIN AND ODEMA (SWELLING)

Edema also known as odema means swelling of body parts due to fluid retention. It is the accumulation of excessive serous fluids in cells or cavities of the body. It mainly affects lower body parts, mostly foot and ankles. It can slow down the healing process, increase the chances of developing skin infection, affect blood circulation and can be painful. Edema is not a disease; it only indicates that something is wrong in the body. Edema is due to an underlying problem in the body. It usually occurs in the feet, ankles and legs, but it can involve your entire body.

Causes of odema(edema) include:

Eating too much salt, Sunburn, Heart failure, Kidney disease, Liver problems from cirrhosis, pregnancy, problems with lymph nodes, especially after mastectomy, Some medicines, standing or walking a lot when the weather is warm.

The symptoms of renal failure include edema, which is an accumulation of fluid characterized by swelling, and a decrease in urination. Other symptoms may include a general ill feeling, exhaustion and headaches. Often, a person with renal failure does not experience any symptoms.

Curcumin attenuates cerebral edema following traumatic brain injury in mice:

In a the Medical College of Georgia a study was made on using curcumin to decrease the water content(odema) resulted from traumatic brain injury.

In a study performed in Taiwan curcumin showed a significant reduction in carrageenan-induced paw edema). Indomethacin inhibited edema by 46.87% and 65.71% at 2 and 3 h after carrageenan injection, respectively.

Many kidney cases used curcumin from kitchen together with the powerful Reno Tech food supplement and after 3 months they got excellent results!!!

Natural Methods of Treating Odema and Swelling:

You can find full details of a natural protocol of treating odema problems in our book:

How to Rid Swelling without Medications which will be printed in the United States.

We can draw the main guidelines of the protocol as follows:

1. Juice that Heal: Noni, Tomato, Cranberry, Aloe Vera and Celery juice can be helpful.

2. Food that Heal: Lettuce, Cucumber, Cabbage and Tomato are also helpful. Pomegranate, Ginger, Almonds and Walnuts and Grape Seed Extract, Baking Powder are well known by their effects on improving odema.

3. Herbs that Heal: Eating 1 tsp of flax seed and black seed every morning for 3 months is good for odema. The Indian herb; Shilajit is one of the best herbs for odema. Dandelion_and_Tribulus terrestris are also very useful.

4. Milk that Heals: Camel milk (as narrated by Prophet Mohammad (PBUH) offers endless health benefits. One of those is treating odema problems. My patients who took 2 glasses of camel milk daily with the food supplement Reno Tech for 3 months found miracle results for both odema and sex!!!!!

5. Herbal Tea that Heals: Hundreds of odema cases who took the herbal tea; Lymph Tea which is simply composed of Celery, Linden and curcumin for 3-6 weeks could easily solve odema problem without medications!!!!!

THE 50 MIRACLE CURES OF CURCUMIN

6. Food Supplemnts that Heal: Many patients obtained excellent results by using the food supplement named: Reno Tech which contains a number of herbs including Curcumin!!!!together with the chlorophyll supplement.

CORIANDER AND PIMPLES, BLACKHEADS AND DRY SKIN

Pimples and blackheads can occur for a variety of reasons, such as bacteria, hormonal fluctuations and excess oil. While there are a variety of different medications available to treat all kinds of acne, you don't have to use such products to clear your skin. With a regular skin care regime and some simple home remedies, you can get rid of pimples and blackheads quickly, without using acne-treatment products.

A teaspoon for coriander juice, mixed with a pinch of turmeric powder, is an effective remedy for pimples, blackheads and dry skin.

Many patients used Curcumin capsules together with our creams, oils and soap in most skin problems including Pimples, Blackheads and Dry Skin and the results were amazing!!!!

We can draw the main guidelines of a protocol as follows:

1. Juice that Heal: Coriander juice (mixed with turmeric powder or mint juice) is used as a treatment for Pimples, Blackheads and Dry Skin: applied to the face in the manner of toner.

2. Food that Heal: Lettuce, Cucumber, Curcumin are also helpful. Apple Cider Vinegar, Baking Powder are well known by their effects on improving Pimples, Blackheads and Dry Skin.

3. Herbs that Heal. Coriander, Aloe Vera: Neem, Turmeric, Papaya., Calendula. Propolis is one of the best herbs for Pimples, Blackheads and Dry Skin.

4. Milk that Heals: Camel milk (as narrated by Prophet Mohammad (PBUH) offers endless health benefits. One of those is treating Pimples, Blackheads and Dry Skin. My patients who took 2 glasses of camel milk daily for 3 weeks found miracle results for Pimples, Blackheads and Dry Skin!!!!!

5. Herbal Tea that Heals: Many Pimples, Blackheads and Dry Skin cases who took our herbal tea composed of Lemon Balm and Coriander seed for 3 weeks could easily solve their Pimples, Blackheads and Dry Skin!

6. Food Supplemnts that Heal:, Vitamin B3, Zinc, MSM together with chlorophyll food supplement.

7. Essential Oils that Heal: Some components of essential oils in turmeric, are excellent antiseptic. In addition, other components have anti microbial and healing effects which have beautiful effects on Pimples, Blackheads and Dry Skin. The oil: Relax U: was successfully used by Pimples, Blackheads and Dry Skin patients!!!

8. Soap that Heals: IRIS Miracle Nano Soap was successfully used by hundreds who got rid of their Pimples, Blackheads and Dry Skin in 7-10 days!!!!

9. Cream that Heals: Many Pimples, Blackheads and Dry Skin patients used Cellu Tech Cream and 14 in One got rid of their Pimples, Blackheads and Dry Skin in 3 weeks.

10. Bath that Heals: Many patients cured their Pimples, Blackheads and Dry Skin by using a 15-minute baking powder bath together with IRIS dead sea salt or mud!!!

CURCUMIN AND PROSTATE HEALTH

The prostate is the male sex gland is the size of a chestnut in the shape of a doughnut through which the urinary tract runs. The prostate is also in charge of discharging sperm during ejaculation semen is mainly made of prostatic fluid. The symptoms of renal failure include edema, which is an accumulation of fluid characterized by swelling, and a decrease in urination. Other symptoms may include a general ill feeling, exhaustion and headaches. Often, a person with renal failure does not experience any symptoms.

Benign prostatic hypertrophy is the gradual enlargement of the prostate it's very a common problem for men more than 50 years of age and 75% of men more than seventy years of age suffer from it. Is cause by hormonal changes in the body as we age, later in life men's production of dihydrotestosterone increases leading to an over production of prostate cells, this makes the prostate grow.

From the phytochemical composition of Turmeric we can notice a number of chemical compounds forming Turmeric act as excellent anti-inflammatory agents, which clearly means that Turmeric is a good candidate to be safely used for prostate health.

Therapeutic potential of curcumin in human prostate cancer showed that curcumin induces apoptosis in both androgen-dependent and androgen-independent prostate cancer cells according to a study performed in Columbia University.

Plant sterols and sterolins – plant sterols are fatty compounds, abundant in seeds, nuts and legumes. It is believed that sterols are active ingredients in saw palmetto and pygeum africanum, which attribute these herbs with their BPH relieving properties. The most abundant plant sterol beta-sitosterol has been currently used in Europe for BPH treatment. In one report, beta-sitosterol was found to induce prostate cancer cell apoptosis (death) in humans. Pytosterols have shown to significantly improve BPH's urological symptoms and urine flow in four double-blind, placebo-controlled studies. Laboratory and animal studies have shown that when plant sterols and sterolins are administrated together, they enhance the immune system and help improve hormonal balance

Many prostate cases used curcumin from kitchen together with the powerful Prosta Tech food supplement and after 3-6 months they got excellent results!!!!!

Triphala – a combination of three fruit extracts: terminalia chebula, terminalia belerica and emblica officinalis. This combination has been used traditionally to improve digestion, elimination and overall body toning. Triphala contains anti-inflammatory, antioxidant and anti-cancerous compounds including tannins, bioflavonoids and vitamin C and is very useful for prostate health.

Natural Methods of Treating Heart Problems:

You can find full details of a natural protocol of treating prostate enlargement in our book:

How to Fix Your Prostate without Medications which will be printed in the United States.

We can draw the main guidelines of the protocol as follows:

1. Juice that Heal: Noni, Tomato, Cranberry, Aloe Vera and Celery juice can be helpful.

THE 50 MIRACLE CURES OF CURCUMIN

2. Food that Heal: Asparagus Soup, Lettuce, Nopal Cactus and Tomato lycopene are also helpful. Garlic is useful to improve the prostate health by the scientific research. Bee Pollens showed remarkable success improving 80% of the cases and curing 40% of them within 6 months, Pomegranate, Baking Powder are well known by their effects on improving prostate health . Pumpkin Seed plays an important role.

3. Herbs that Heal: Eating 1 tsp of curcumin and black seed every morning for 3 months is good for Prostate. The Indian herb; Shilajit is one of the best herbs for prostate. Corn Silk, Uva Ursi, Myrrh, Milk Thistle, Neem, Dandelion, Goldenseal, Saw Palmetto and Tribulus terrestris, Guggul, Nettle Root, Sandalwood are also very useful.

4. Milk that Heals: Camel milk (as narrated by Prophet Mohammad (PBUH) offers endless health benefits. One of those is treating prostate problems. My patients who took 2 glasses of camel milk daily with the food supplement Prosta Tech for 3-6 months found miracle results for both prostate and sex!!!!!

5. Herbal Tea that Heals: Hundreds of kidney cases who took the herbal tea; Pros Tea which is simply composed of Corn Silk, Crataeva nurvala and curcumin for 3-6 months could easily improve prostate health!!!

6. Food Supplemnts that Heal: Many patients obtained excellent results by using the food supplement named: Prosta Tech which contains a number of herbs including curcumin!! together with chlorophyll supplement.

CURCUMIN AND PROSTATITIS

The prostate is the male sex gland is the size of a chestnut in the shape of a doughnut through which the urinary tract runs. The prostate is also in charge of discharging sperm during ejaculation semen is mainly made of prostatic fluid.

Prostatitis is an inflammation in the prostate gland; this is a very common problem for men of all ages. Bacteria from different parts of the body infect the prostate and that causes prostatitis. Once infected the prostate swells restricting the flow of urine and causing urine retention. There are three types of prostatitis: acute infectious prostatitis, chronic infectious prostatitis, and noninfectious prostatitis

From the phytochemical composition of turmeric we can notice a number of chemical compounds forming turmeric act as excellent anti-inflammatory agents, which clearly means that coriander is a good candidate to be safely used for prostatitis.

Turmeric serves both as an herb and a spice. It is a healing herb that is used effectively in different parts of the globe. While Indians use it for its anti-inflammatory properties, many other nations use this perennial herb for prostatitis

Many prostatitis cases used turmeric from kitchen together with the powerful Prosta Tech food supplement and after 3-6 months they got excellent results!!!

Natural Methods of Treating Prostatitis Problems:

You can find full details of a natural protocol of treating prostatitis in our book:

How to Fix Prostatitis without Medications which will be printed in the United States.

We can draw the main guidelines of the protocol as follows:

1. **Juice that Heal:** Radish, Pomegranate, Tomato, Cranberry, Aloe Vera and Celery juice can be helpful.

2. **Food that Heal:** Asparagus Soup, Nopal Cactus, Cabbage and Tomato lycopene are also helpful. Garlic is useful to improve the prostatitis by the scientific research.

3. **Herbs that Heal:** Eating 1 tsp of flax seed and black seed every morning for 3 months is good for Prostatitis. The Indian herb ; Shilajit is one of the best herbs for prostatitis.Corn Silk, Uva Ursi, Myrrh, Milk Thistle, Neem, Dandelion, Goldenseal, Saw Palmetto and Tribulus terrestris, Guggul, Nettle Root, Sandalwood are also very useful.

4. **Milk that Heals:** Camel milk (as narrated by Prophet Mohammad (PBUH) offers endless health benefits. One of those is treating prostate problems. My patients who took 2 glasses of camel milk daily with the food supplement Prosta Tech for 3-6 months found miracle results for both prostatitis and sex!!!!!

5. **Herbal Tea that Heals:** Hundreds of prostatitis cases who took the herbal tea ;Pros Tea which is simply composed of Corn Silk, Crataeva nurvala and Coriander seed for 3-6 months could easily improve heart functions!!

6. **Food Supplemnts that Heal:** Many patients obtained excellent results by using the food supplement named: Prosta Tech which contains a number of herbs including turmeric, Amla berries'

7. **Vitamins that Heal**: Vitamin B17, Vitamin C, Zinc and Vitamin E

8. **Magnet that Heals**: While most of chemical and herbal formulas failed to cure prostatitis my patients were successful in curing their prostatitis by using the Russian Magnetic Prostate Rod after 13 years of continuous usage of antibiotics. For details please refer to our book: **How to Fix Your Prostatitis without Medications** .

CURCUMIN AND PSORIASIS

Major Causes of Psoriasis

Psoriasis is considered a non-curable, long-term (chronic) skin condition. It has a variable course, periodically improving and worsening. Sometimes psoriasis may clear for years and stay in remission. Some people have worsening of their symptoms in the colder winter months. Many people report improvement in warmer months, climates, or with increased sunlight exposure especially the balanced UV layer found in the Dead Sea area in Jordan and Palestine.

Following is a list of causes or underlying that could possibly cause Psoriasis includes: Genetic predisposition, Factors that may aggravate psoriasis include stress, excessive alcohol consumption, and smoking, Withdrawal of systemic steroids, Drugs, including salicylates, iodine, lithium, phenylbutazone, oxyphenbutazone, trazodone, penicillin, hydroxychloroquine, calcipotriol, interferon-alpha, and interferon-beta injection strong, irritating topical, including tar, anthralin, steroids under occlusion, and zinc pyrithione in shampoo, Infections, Sunlight or phototherapy, Cholestatic jaundice, Calcium deficiency, Sudden withdrawal of oral corticosteroids (prednisone).

It has been found that psoriasis patients suffer from folic acid and Vitamin B12 deficiency.

Coal tar *is probably the oldest psoriasis remedy known to medicine and its origins as an anti- psoriasis treatment but it is famous with its bad reputation to cause skin cancer!!!*

Some famous products in the market use Salicylic acid inside creams but it causes many side effects and skin irritation!!!!

Curcumin serves both as an herb and a spice. It is a healing herb that is used effectively in different parts of the globe. While Indians use it for its anti-inflammatory properties, many other nations use this perennial herb for psoriasis.

Natural Methods of Treating Psoriasis:

You can find full details of a natural protocol of treating psoriasis problems in our book:

How to Rid Psoriasis in 4 Weeks without Medications which will be printed in the United States.

We can draw the main guidelines of the protocol as follows:

1. Juice that Heal: Coriander juice (mixed with turmeric powder or mint juice) is used as a treatment for psoriasis as a drink, and applied to the psoriasis areas.

2. Food that Heal: Lettuce, Cucumber, Curcumin are also helpful. Apple Cider Vinegar, Baking Powder is well known by their effects on improving psoriasis.

3. Herbs that Heal. Coriander, Aloe Vera: Neem, Turmeric, Papaya., Calendula. Propolis is one of the best herbs for psoriasis.

4. Milk that Heals: Camel milk (as narrated by Prophet Mohammad (PBUH) offers endless health benefits. One of those is treating psoriasis. My patients who took 2 glasses of camel milk daily for 4 weeks found miracle results for psoriasis!!!!!

5. Herbal Tea that Heals: Hundreds of psoriasis cases who took the herbal tea composed of Turmeric and Coriander seed for 4 weeks together with the cream; Psoria Tech(IRIS PS) did easily solve their psoriasis without medications!!and one of the difficult cases was a female medical doctor who suffered for several years of her severe Rheumatic Psoriasis and finally got rid of both Rheumatoid and Psoriasis!!!

THE 50 MIRACLE CURES OF CURCUMIN

6. Food Supplemnts that Heal:, Vitamin B3, Zinc, MSM together with chlorophyll food supplement.

7. Essential Oils that Heal: Some of component of essential oils in turmeric, is an excellent antiseptic. In addition, other components have anti microbial and healing effects which do not let psoriasis go worse.

8. Soap that Heals: IRIS Miracle Nano Soap was successfully used by hundreds who got rid of their psoriasis in 4 weeks!!!!

9. Cream that Heals: Many psoriasis patients used the Psoria Tech Cream which is very powerful to rid of psoriasis in 4-6 weeks.

10. Bath that Heals: Many patients cured their psoriasis by using a 15-minute baking powder bath together with the Dead Sea mud!!!

CURCUMIN AND SEX

From the phytochemical composition of turmeric we can notice a number of chemical compounds forming turmeric act as vasodilator agents, which clearly means that turmeric is a good candidate to be safely used for sex.

Who would think that you could help cure a low sex drive with curcumin? Of course you should always consult your physician if you have any ongoing sexual dysfunction, but curcumin can be a quick fix. It's natural and healthy with no side effects typically associated with Erectile Dysfunction prescription medication.

The Middle Ages, there was a drink that was created by Hippocrates that became a staple at many wedding parties. It contains several herbs such as curcumin, cardamom, clove, ginger, coriander and cinnamon. This drink is called **"Hippocras"**. This drink was eventually banned because it stimulated the libido too much. Now you can create and drink this drink yourself to help cure a low sex drive.

Natural Methods of Treating Hypertension:

You can find full details of a natural protocol of treating sex impotence in our book:

How to be a Real Man without Medications which will be printed in the United States.

We can draw the main guidelines of the protocol as follows:

1. Juice that Heal: Acai, Strawberry, Tomato, and Celery juice can be helpful.

2. Food that Heal: Banana and Potato (rich in potassium), Cocoa, Dark Chocolate, Yogurt and Apple are also helpful... Honey and Cinnamon are useful for low sex drive by the scientific research.

3. **Herbs that Heal:** Eating 1 tsp of celery seed and flax seed every morning for 3 months is said to prevent hypertension due to heredity factors.

4. **Milk that Heals:** Camel milk (as narrated by Prophet Mohammad (PBUH) offers endless health benefits. One of those is treating impotence and infertility. Camel milk is said to be the **Viagra of the Future**". My patients who took 2 glasses of camel milk daily with the food supplement: Camel Tech for 3 months found miracle results for sex!!!!!

5. **Herbal Tea that Heals:** Hundreds of low libido cases who took the herbal tea ;Heart & Love Tea which is simply composed of Hibiscus, Cinnamon, Mint and Coriander seed for 3-6 months could easily restore their sexual power to normal!!!

6. **Food Supplemnts that Heal:** Many patients obtained excellent results by using the food supplemensts named: ViaTech and Vita-X which contain a number of stimulating herbs including Curcumin!!!!Bee Pollen is important too.

Hippocras Sex Drink

- 3/4 Gallon Grape juice
- 1 Cup Honey
- 2 Tablespoons cinnamon
- 2 Tablespoons Fresh Grated Ginger
- 1 Tablespoon Nutmeg
- 1 Tablespoon Mace
- 1 Tablespoon Cloves
- 1 Tablespoon Cardamom
- 1 Tablespoon Coriander
- 1 Tablespoon Cayenne
- 1 Tablespoon Curcumin

Mix all spices together and set aside. Heat the grape juice to just below boiling. Add spices to the juice and allow cooling. Pour the mix into air tight glass containers and set it in a cool dark place for one week. Strain the juice and return to air tight containers. Let this concoction rest for about one month before drinking. It will keep unopened for years, about four days after opening.

CURCUMIN AND SMALLPOX

From World Health Organization (WHO): Smallpox is an acute contagious disease caused by variola virus.

Smallpox, which is believed to have originated over 3, 000 years ago in India or Egypt, is one of the most devastating diseases known to humanity. For centuries, repeated epidemics swept across continents, decimating populations and changing the course of history. In some ancient cultures, smallpox was such a major killer of infants that custom forbade the naming of a newborn until the infant had caught the disease and proved it would survive.

Smallpox killed Queen Mary II of England, Emperor Joseph I of Austria, King Luis I of Spain, Tsar Peter II of Russia, Queen Ulrika Elenora of Sweden, and King Louis XV of France.

The disease, for which no effective treatment was ever developed, killed as many as 30% of those infected. Between 65–80% of survivors were marked with deep pitted scars (pockmarks), most prominent on the face. Blindness was another complication. In 18th century Europe, a third of all reported cases of blindness were due to smallpox.

One teaspoon fresh coriander/curcumin juice, mixed with 1 or 2 seeds of banana, given once daily regularly, for a week is a very effective preventive measure against small pox. It is believed that putting fresh leaf juice in the eyes, during an attack of small pox, prevents eye damage.

Eating curcumin promotes a faster curing process when suffering from smallpox while reducing the pain simultaneously.

Egyptians used Henna to treat smallpox.

Turmeric was successfully used to rid of smallpox and chickenpox.

The Herbs that are famous to treat smallpox are: Garlic, Bistort, Black Cohosh, Goldenseal, Hyssop, Lobelia, Tansy And Yarrow.

The cream; All in One is very useful for smallpox well as gangrene ad fungus.

The oil mix of Lavender and Coriander are very useful too.

CURCUMIN AND SORE THROAT

Sore throats are one of the most common reasons why people see a doctor. In the United States, sore throats account for more than 18 million visits to the doctor each year.

One of the easiest, least expensive home remedies to treat a sore throat is the following herbal formula:

1 ½ cups of water

1 table spoon of Coriander seed OR curcumin

Directions:

1-Soak coriander/curcumin inside water over night.

2-Discard coriander seed(or Curcumin) next morning.

3-Gargle with water and let it reach inside your throat

4-Throw water away.You will feel better in less than 1 hour.

5-Repeat the same process many times till you are OK.

Other home remedies:

Gargle with salty water many times till symptoms disappear.

Use Zinc, Elderberry, Grapefruit seed extract, garlic

Use Bee Propolis which is equivalent to 132 antibiotics.

Uses our oil mix RELAX U externally.

Slippery Elm, Licorice, Hyssop, Elecampane, Ginger, Marshmallow, Honey Water, and Sage.

CURCUMIN AND TRIGLYCERIDES

Triglycerides are the chemical form in which most fat exists in food as well as in the body. They're also present in blood plasma and, in association with cholesterol, form the plasma lipids.

Triglycerides in plasma are derived from fats eaten in foods or made in the body from other energy sources like carbohydrates. Calories ingested in a meal and not used immediately by tissues are converted to triglycerides and transported to fat cells to be stored. Hormones regulate the release of triglycerides from fat tissue so they meet the body's needs for energy between meals.

Everyone with high triglycerides needs to keep it under control, but it may be even more important for some groups of people, such as

- People with a family history of early heart disease
- People with high blood pressure
- People with diabetes
- People with obesity
- People with continuous stress
- Males over age 45
- Females over age 55
- Smokers

From the phytochemical composition of turmeric we can notice a number of chemical compounds forming turmeric act as anti-lipid and anti- triglycerides agents, which clearly means that coriander is a good candidate to be safely used for high triglycerides.

Curcumin serves both as an herb and a spice. It is a healing herb that is used effectively in different parts of the globe. While Indians use it for its anti-inflammatory properties, many other nations use this perennial herb for high cholesterol and triglycerides.

Curcumin was given to rats that had been fed a high-fat and high-triglycerides diet. The spice lowered total cholesterol and triglycerides significantly!!

Cardiovascular Disease and Blood Lipids
Curcumin lowers cholesterol and triglyceride levels, helping to reduce the risk of atherosclerosis and thereby heart attack and stroke. It does this through two mechanisms: by inhibiting the uptake of these lipids in the intestines, and by enhancing their breakdown and excretion.

In for high triglyceride management it has been shown that Curcumin acts as an anti-lipid agent and also helps in the vasodilatation of veins!!

Many high cholesterol cases used Curcumin from kitchen together with the powerful Choles Tech food supplement and after 3 months they got excellent results!!!

Natural Methods of Treating High Triglyceride:

You can find full details of a natural protocol of treating high triglyceride in our book:

How to Lower Your High Triglyceride to Normal without Medications which will be printed in the United States.

We can draw the main guidelines of the protocol as follows:

1. Juice that Heal: Acai, Tomato, Cucumber, and Celery juice can be helpful.

2. Food that Heal: Dark Chocolate, Peanut Butter, Lettuce, Cucumber, Sunflower seeds, Yogurt and Tomato are also helpful. Garlic is useful to lower the blood high triglyceride by the scientific research. Apple cider vinegar to lower triglyceride: It is said that an 8oz. apple juice with a tablespoon of apple cider vinegar will lower cholesterol and triglyceride. Almonds and Walnuts are very famous for lowering triglyceride. Grape Seed Extract is well known by its

THE 50 MIRACLE CURES OF CURCUMIN

effect in lowering triglyceride. Royal Jelly is a beautiful food to lower triglyceride.

3. Herbs that Heal: Eating 1 tsp of Curcumin, flax seed and black seed every morning for 3 months is said to prevent high triglyceride due to heredity factors. They also cure high triglyceride due to obesity, as both seeds have weight reducing properties. The Indian famous herb; Guggul is also useful.

4. Milk that Heals: Camel milk (as narrated by Prophet Mohammad (PBUH) offers endless health benefits. One of those is treating high triglyceride. Camel milk is said to be the vasodilator of the Future". My patients who took 2 glasses of camel milk daily with the food supplement: CholesTech for 3 months found miracle results for both high triglyceride and sex!!!!!

5. Herbal Tea that Heals: Hundreds of high triglyceride cases who took the herbal tea ;Heart & Love Tea which is simply composed of Cinnamon, Fenugreek and Curcumin for 3-6 months could easily reduce their high cholesterol to normal!!!

6. Food Supplements that Heal: Many patients obtained excellent results by using the food supplement named: Choles Tech which contains a number of anti-lipid herbs including Curcumin!!!!

7.Exercise that Heals: One of the most important factors that helped thousands of people to reduce high triglyceride is to perform daily exercise together with Royal Jelly and L-LYSINE amino acid from health stores.

The 1992 Indian Journal of Physiology reported that ten human volunteers taking curcumin showed a 29% increase in beneficial HDL cholesterol in only 7 days. Total cholesterol also fell 11.6% and **lipid peroxidation was reduced by 33%.**

In a study involving rats fed a high-fat diet (30% of calories from fat), treatment with curcumin, capsaicin, or the combination of the two dietary spice compounds, was found to **reduce elevated**

triglycerides (by 12-20%), total cholesterol, and lipid peroxide levels.

CURCUMIN AND ULCER

Peptic ulcer disease refers to painful sores or ulcers in the lining of the stomach or first part of the small intestine, called the duodenum.

What Causes Ulcers?

No single cause has been found for ulcers. However, it is now clear that an ulcer is the end result of an imbalance between digestive fluids in the stomach and duodenum. Ulcers can be caused by:

- Infection with a type of bacteria called Helicobacter pylori **(H. Pylori)** which also causes **stomach cancer!!!**

- Use of chemical painkillers steroidal anti-inflammatory drugs (NSAIDs). Even aspirin coated with a special substance can still cause ulcers.

Excess acid production from gastrinomas, tumors of the acid producing cells of the stomach that increases acid output.

Curcumin helps cure ulcer, inflammation and spasm.

As for drinks, one should avoid alcoholic drinks completely.

Curcumin serves both as an herb and a spice. It is a healing herb that is used effectively in different parts of the globe. While Indians use it for its anti-inflammatory properties, many other nations use this perennial herb for peptic ulcer.

As for drinks, one should avoid alcoholic drinks completely.

Natural Methods of Treating Ulcer:

You can find full details of a natural protocol of treating peptic ulcer problems in our book:

How to Fix Ulcer without Medications which will be printed in the United States soon.

We can draw the main guidelines of the protocol as follows:

1. Juice that Heal: Licorice, Cabbage juice represents a miracle cure for ulcer.

2. Food that Heal: Cherry, Lettuce, Cucumber, Cabbage are also helpful. Pomegranate, Ginger, Almonds, Walnuts, Baking Powder are well known by their effects on improving peptic ulcer.

3. Herbs that Heal: Eating 1 tsp of Fenugreek, Aloe Vera, Ginger, Lemon Balm, Chamomile, Peppermint, Licorice and Curcumin every morning for 3 weeks is good for mouth ulcer. The Indian herb; Shilajit is one of the best herbs for peptic ulcer.

4. Milk that Heals: Camel milk (as narrated by Prophet Mohammad (PBUH) offers endless health benefits. One of those is treating peptic ulcer. My patients who took 2 glasses of camel milk daily for 3 months found miracle results for both peptic ulcer and sex!!!!!

5. Herbal Tea that Heals: Hundreds of mouth ulcer cases who took the herbal tea ;Diges Tech Tea which is simply composed of Licorice, Alfalfa, Pomegranate Peels, Propolis and Curcumin for 3 weeks could easily solve their peptic ulcer

6. Food Supplemnts that Heal: Many patients obtained excellent results by using the food supplement named: Stomach Care which contains a number of herbs including Curcumin!!!! together with the chlorophyll supplement.

CURCUMIN AND URINARY TRACT INFECTION (UTI)

Urinary Tract Infection (UTI) is an infection by the bacteria of the urinary tract which includes kidney, ureterus, bladder or urethra. This bacterium enters the opening of the urethra and procreates in the urinary tract causing urinary tract infection. This can be very painful and a major cause of distress in your life. If it is not contained in the earlier stages it is likely to spread to your kidneys, which can become a serious health issue. The infection of the bladder can develop into cystitis- a very common problem faced by women. Urinary Tract Infection can infect anyone but women are more susceptible to this disease. Children too suffer from this disorder but the headcount is very low in comparison to adults. Sexual intercourse is another reason for urinary tract infection.

From the phytochemical composition of turmeric we can notice a number of chemical compounds forming coriander act as excellent anti-inflammatory agents, which clearly means that coriander is a good candidate to be safely used for UTI!!

Curcumin serves both as an herb and a spice. It is a healing herb that is used effectively in different parts of the globe. While Indians use it for its anti-inflammatory properties, and hence for UTI.

Many stories about using Curcumin as anti-inflammatory tool for **UTI!!!!** Many Qatari and Saudi UTI patients; got rid of it within 4 weeks only!!!!After starting taking coriander tea together with the food supplement URI TECH and Cranberry Juice without any medications!!!!!

Natural Methods of Treating UTI Problems:

You can find full details of a natural protocol of treating UTI problems in our book:

How to Rid UTI in 3 Weeks without Medications which will be printed in the United States.

We can draw the main guidelines of the protocol as follows:

1. Juice that Heal: Cranberry and 2-3 glasses water on empty stomach can be very helpful.

2. Food that Heal: Lettuce, Cucumber, Cabbage are also helpful. Pomegranate, Baking Powder is well known by **their** effects on improving UTI.

3. Herbs that Heal: Eating 1 tsp of corn silk and cinnamon with honey every morning for 3 weeks is good for UTI. The Indian herb; Shilajit is one of the best herbs for UTI._Dandelion and Tribulus terrestris are also useful.

4. Milk that Heals: Camel milk (as narrated by Prophet Mohammad (PBUH) offers endless health benefits. One of those is treating UTI problems. My patients who took 2 glasses of camel milk daily with the food supplement Uri Tech for 3 months found miracle results for both UTI and sex!!!!!

5. Herbal Tea that Heals: Hundreds of UTI cases who took the herbal tea; Uri Tech Tea which is simply composed of Corn Silk, Parsley, Curcumin and Coriander seed for 3-6 weeks could solve their UTI problem without medications!!!!!

6. Food Supplemnts that Heal: Many patients obtained excellent results by using the food supplement named: Uri Tech which contains a number of herbs including Curcumin!!!! together with **the** chlorophyll supplement.

CURCUMIN AND WEIGHT LOSS

Being overweight is a common condition, especially where food supplies are plentiful and lifestyles are sedentary. As much as 64% of the United States adult population is considered either overweight or obese, and this percentage has increased over the last four decades.

Excess weight has reached epidemic proportions globally, with more than 1 billion adults being either overweight or obese Increases have been observed across all age groups.

Causes

Factors which may contribute to this imbalance include:

- Limited physical exercise
- Overeating
- Poor nutrition
- Genetic predisposition
- Hormonal imbalances (e.g. hypothyroidism)
- Metabolic disorders, Eating disorders
- Alcoholism
- Stress
- Insufficient or poor-quality sleep
- Psychotropic medication
- Smoking cessation

In some cases, insulin dependent diabetes can cause weight gain in some sufferers, as opposed to type II diabetes which mostly comes on as a result of being overweight.

Natural Methods of Treating Obesity Problems:

You can find full details of a natural protocol of treating heart problems in our book: **How to be Slim without Medications** which will be printed in the United States soon.

We can draw the main guidelines of the protocol as follows:

1. Juice that Heal: Tomato, Cranberry, Cabbage and Celery juice can be helpful.

2. Food that Heal: Asparagus Soup, Lettuce, Cucumber, Cabbage and Tomato are also helpful. Yogurt, Ginger, Almonds and Sunflower and Grape Seed Extract, Baking Powder are well known by their effects on losing weight.

3. Herbs that Heal: Eating 1 tsp of flax seed and cinnamon every morning for 3 months is good for obesity. The Indian herb; Shilajit is one of the best herbs for obesity. Dandelion, Anise, Senna, Caralluma Fimbriata and Licorice are also very useful.

4. Milk that Heals: Camel milk (as narrated by Prophet Mohammad (PBUH) offers endless health benefits. One of those is treating obesity problems. My patients who took 2 glasses of camel milk daily with the food supplement Slim Tech for 3 months found miracle results for both obesity and sex!!!!!

5. Herbal Tea that Heals: Hundreds of obesity cases who took the herbal tea ;Dr.Slim Tea which is simply composed of Anise, Fennel, Senna and Curcumin for 3-6 months could easily reduce weight without medications!!!!!

6. Food Supplemnts that Heal: Many patients obtained excellent results by using the food supplement named: Slim Tech which contains a number of herbs including Curcumin!!! together with kelp food supplement.

CORIANDER AS AN EFFICIENT HEAVY METALS DETOX

An efficient liver detoxification system is vital to health and in order to support this process it is essential that many key nutrients are included in the diet. Vitamins and minerals – particularly the B vitamins. Cytochrome P450 is induced by some toxins and by some foods and nutrients. Drugs and environmental toxins activate P450 to combat their destructive effects, and in so doing, not only use up compounds needed for this detoxification system but contribute significantly to free radical formation and oxidative stress. Curcumin inhibits phase I while *stimulating* phase II. This effect can be very useful in preventing certain types of cancer. **Curcumin** has been found to inhibit carcinogens, such as *benzopyrene* (found in charcoal-broiled meat), from inducing cancer.

Glutathione is also an important antioxidant. This combination of detoxification and free radical protection, results in glutathione being one of the most important anticarcinogens and antioxidants in our cells.

There is a long list of plants which exert beneficial effects on liver function. However, the most impressive research has been done on *silymarin*, the flavonoids extracted from *silybum marianum* (milk thistle).

Delicious recipe for heavy-metal cleansing:

CORIANDER CHELATION PESTO

4 cloves garlic
1/3 cup Brazil nuts (selenium)
1/3 cup sunflower seeds (cysteine)
1/3 cup pumpkin seeds (zinc, magnesium)
2 cups packed fresh coriander (cilantro, Chinese parsley)
2/3 cup flaxseed oil
4 tablespoons lemon juice (vitamin C)

2 tsp dulse powder
Sea salt to taste
Process the coriander and flaxseed oil in a blender until the coriander is chopped. Add the garlic, nuts and seeds, dulse and lemon juice and mix until the mixture is finely blended into a paste. Add a pinch to sea salt to taste and blend again. Store in dark glass jars if possible. It freezes well, so purchase coriander in season and fill jars to last through the year.

Coriander has been proven to **chelate toxic metals from our bodies** in a relatively short period of time. Combined with the benefits of the other ingredients, this recipe is a powerful tissue cleanser. Two teaspoons of this pesto daily for three weeks is purportedly enough to increase the **urinary excretion of mercury, lead and aluminum**, thus effectively removing these toxic metals from our bodies. We can consider doing this cleanses for three weeks at least once a year. The pesto is delicious on toast, baked potatoes, and pasta.

Another effective heavy metals detox formula is:

2 ml(2 droppers full or 52 drops) contains:

· 50 mgs. - Nanocolloidal cell wall decimated **Chlorella Pyrenoidosa**

.12 mls. - Nanocolloidal Cilantro

· 10 mgs. - Nanocolloidal *PolyFlor

· 75 mgs/liter nanocolloidal Silica

CURCUMIN CABBAGE MIRACLE SLIMMING SOUP

Ingredients: (This soup is famous for its slimming miracle results):

450g onions
1/2 Savoy cabbage (about 400g)
2 tablespoons olive oil
2 red or 4 green chillies, finely chopped
4 garlic cloves, finely chopped
About 5 cm fresh root ginger, peeled and chopped
2 tablespoons curcumin(curry)powder.
800ml good vegetable stock
400ml tin of coconut milk
Bunch of fresh coriander, chopped
Juice of 3 limes
Salt and black pepper.

Finely chop the onions and very finely shred the cabbage, either by hand or by using the finest slicing disc on a food processor. Heat the oil in a pan, add the onion and cabbage, and cook them over a moderate heat for a couple of minutes before adding the chillies, garlic, ginger and curcumin. Continue cooking for about 5 minutes, stirring regularly, until the onion and cabbage are tender but still have a bite to them.

Bring the stock to the boil in a separate pan and add to the vegetables. Simmer for 5 minutes, then add the coconut milk, half of the fresh coriander, the lime juice and finally salt and pepper. Serve the soup with extra coriander to taste.

Why Curcumin is Effective for Weight Loss?

It's unclear what accounted for curcumin's effect on weight loss in different studies. It's thought that it may interfere with one of the enzymes needed for building fat tissue. Some studies have also shown that curcumin lowers insulin resistance, thereby decreasing the risk of type 2 diabetes. The ability to lower insulin resistance may also partially account for its ability to promote fat loss.

Curcumin, the natural pigment that gives the spice turmeric its yellow colour, may prevent reduce body weight gain, and help in the fight against obesity, suggests new data from a study with mice.

A Tufts University study has found that curcumin, a polyphenol found in turmeric, has shown promise as a weight loss aid...in mice.

Curcumin, the major polyphenol found in turmeric, appears to reduce weight gain in mice and suppress the growth of fat tissue in mice and cell models. Researchers at the Jean Mayer USDA Human Nutrition Research Center on Aging at Tufts University (USDA HNRCA) studied mice fed high fat diets supplemented with Curcumin.

CURCUMIN, LICE AND DANDRUFF

Head **lice** are tiny insects that live on the scalp. They can be spread by close contact with other people. These lice only live in hair and occasionally eyebrows and eyelashes.

Dandruff is a form of dermatitis caused by fungal infection of the skin and hair follicles. Dandruff is also known as Seborrheic Dermatitis, Cradle Cap, Seborrhea and Seborrheic eczema. Dandruff is characterized by scaly skin which is shed in the form of flakes. Dandruff if not treated can lead to loss of hair and eye infections. Guava fruit extract is very effective in the treatment of dandruff. Regular application of Guava fruit extract helps to cure dandruff. Guava fruit extracts are a natural alternative to commonly used as anti-fungus.

Turmeric oil/Coriander oil is one of the best remedies to kill lice on head.

Turmeric oil/Coriander oil is one of the best solutions for dandruff problems and it is included in our **Magic Hair Oil** and **Smart Shampoo**.

Other Effective Home Remedies for dandruff:

Henna pasted with water and applied on scalp.

Coconut, Pineapple and Lime: Grated coconut and pineapple and mixed thoroughly with lime (squeeze it) and coconut water. Then sieved and used to wash the hair every five days.

5 to 10 Guava fruits crushed into a fine paste. And applied twice daily for a week. The Dandruff is resolved in a week.

Neem oil is used after shampoo on daily basis. It is good for both lice and dandruff.

Spinach infused in water over night and then used twice daily till dandruff is cured.

Lime juice is rinsed on hair twice daily.

Apple Cider Vinegar is mixed with our shampoo to cure dandruff.

Olive Oil is very helpful to treat dandruff.

Olive Oil mixed with Almond oil is fast in curing dandruff.

Tea Tree Oil is also helpful to treat dandruff.

Aloe Vera Gel is used for 10 minutes on scalp and then washed by shampoo.

For head lice problem wash your hair with vinegar. It will kill all the nits in two days. Apply coconut oil to your head after shampoo and condition. Add ten to fifteen drops of tea tree oil into shampoo bottle and use it daily. This will kill all the lice. Massage your head with mayonnaise and comb it after 2 hours. This will kill all the lice and their eggs. Apply a mixture of lemon and butter on your head, wait for 15 seconds and then rinse your head.

Camphor oil and Lemon oil are excellent for lice treatment.

The Oil:Lice Tech Oil is very fast in killing lice in minutes.

CURCUMIN, NAUSEA AND VOMITING

Nausea and vomiting are not diseases, but rather are symptoms of many different conditions, such as infection ("stomach flu"), food poisoning, motion sickness, overeating, blocked intestine, illness, concussion or brain injury, appendicitis, and migraines. Nausea and vomiting can sometimes be symptoms of more serious diseases such as heart attacks, kidney or liver disorders, central nervous system disorders, brain tumors, and some forms of cancer.

Curcumin with Ginger cure nausea and tendency to vomit: Boiled curcumin water with sugar candy is beneficial. Vomiting during pregnancy can also be treated.

Home remedies for nausea and vomiting:

Effective home remedy for vomiting using Cauliflower: It contains alkaline substances which purify blood. Eating cooked or raw cauliflower is **beneficial in bloody vomiting.** The patients of TB should definitely take it.

Natural home remedy for vomiting using Mint leaves: Take half a cup of the juice of mint leaves at an interval of every two hours. You can add lemon juice to it. Frequent use of curcumin, ginger and mint is quite beneficial for vomiting.

Herbal home remedy for vomiting using Neem: Grind 25 gms. Of neem leaves, mix with water, strain and drink. It can check all types of vomiting.

Simple home remedy for vomiting: Vomiting during pregnancy- soak 50 gms. Rice in 250 ml. water. After half an hour put 5 gms. Coriander seeds in it. Then after ten minutes stir and strain. Take them as four doses in one day. It will provide relief to the pregnant woman from vomiting.

Good home remedy for vomiting: Grind two cloves and give it with honey to the pregnant woman, in case of vomiting. Sucking a roasted clove treats vomiting. Whenever vomiting takes place, suck a roasted clove.

Effective home remedy for vomiting: Soak ripe tamarind in water, then mash, strain and drink it. It will check vomiting.

Diet tips for vomiting

Banana: Eating ripe bananas checks bloody vomiting.

Pistachio: Eating four pistachios will vomiting and nausea.

Harad: Taking harad mixed with honey controls vomiting.

Honey: Onion juice mixed with honey checks vomiting.

Water-melon: In case of heart burn after meals and yellowish vomit, take water-melon juice with sugar candy.

Onion: Taking 2 tsp. of the mixed juice of ginger and onion can control vomiting.

Sugarcane: In case of bilious vomiting, taking sugarcane juice mixed with honey will be beneficial.

Cinnamon: Take cinnamon powder mixed with honey to get relief from bilious vomiting.

Basil: The juice of basil leaves checks vomiting. Taking honey mixed with the juice of basil leaves provides relief from vomiting and nausea.

CURCUMIN IN PERFUMES, FLAVORS & NATURAL DYE INDUSTRY

Turmeric oil is obtained by steam distillation of turmeric leaves. It is mainly cultivated in India.

Turmeric oil is an essential composition in many perfumes and cologne famous names; for example:

Turmeric oil is used in one of the 10 top fragrances in india:

> **Fragrance personality:** *Turmeric and Roses*
>
> The tropical rhizome, turmeric, is valued in India not only for the beautiful saffron-yellow color it gives to culinary preparations, but also for its antiseptic, purifying purposes. The haldi ceremony, in which the bride and the groom are rubbed with turmeric and sandalwood.

Turmeric is used in food and drink flavoring and here is an example of one of the new mixes:

Curry Flavor, Anise Oil, Clove, Coriander, Cumin, Cinnamon, Ginger, Black Pepper, Turmeric Palm, Capsicum.

Ayurvedic Bar Soap, Sandal-Tumeric

History and Usage: This Ayurvedic soap is made in India from all natural oils and herbal extracts, according to Ayurvedic formulas that were created to help clear-up different skin conditions: Sandal-Turmeric: Recommended for blemished skin, normal to oily skin and Pitta-Kapha type constitution. For generations in India, a simple paste of sandalwood and turmeric has been applied to the facial skin to preserve youth and a flawless complexion.

Turmeric Yellow Extracts is started to be used in Natural Dye Industry:for example:

The country's natural dye industry makes a breakthrough as the common service facility (CSF) on natural dye extraction and application in Aklan is now into full commercial scale, the

Philippine Textile Research Institute (PTRI) announced recently. They extract the natural yellow color, golden yellow, greenish yellow, and yellow orange colors from the Rhizomes of turmeric.

Turmeric Ice Cream Secret Formula

Turmeric Ice Cream - Recipe: Serves 6

It also recently occured to me that Semifreddo is the best thing to make if you don't have an ice cream maker. It is very simple, beautiful to serve and sounds fancy:
1. Get together 5 or 6 oz. of fresh Turmeric root.
2. Change into all black clothing.
3. Peel Turmeric.
4. Place into a small food processor or blender with 1/2 c. of milk and puree.
5. Pour 2 cups of milk, 3/4 cups of sugar (more or less depending on how sweet you like your ice cream) and 2 scrambled eggs into a sauce pan.
6. Heat and stir over med. low. Do not allow the mixture to boil or you'll end up with milk sweet scambled eggs. Just stir more or less constantly for 10 minutes.
7. Put in the fridge or freezer to chill
8. Whip 2 cups of cream to peaks.
9. Once everything is cold, put it all into an ice cream maker for 20 minutes.

Turmeric Semifreddo: Serves 6
1. Separate 3 eggs.
2. Beat the egg yolks with 1/2 c. of caster sugar until they turn pale yellow.
3. Beat the egg whites until they come to stiff peaks.
4. Whip 1.5 cups of heavy cream to peaks.
5. Put on all black clothing
6. Peel 5-6 oz. of fresh Turmeric root.
7. Puree with 1/2 cup of milk in a food processor or blender.
8. Line a loaf pan or any type of mold with plastic wrap.
9. Gently add the Turmeric to the egg yolk mixture.
10. Gently fold the egg yolks into the whipped cream and egg whites.
11. When combined, pour into mold, cover with plastic wrap and freeze overnight.

Turmeric SunScreen Nano Cream

Turmeric, also called Indian saffron, is not only a popular culinary herb in some cuisines, but is an important herb in Ayurvedic medicine. It grows widely throughout India, Asia and parts of Africa. Turmeric cream has been used for centuries by Hindu women who prize light, glowing skin, especially for special events such as weddings. Chemically, turmeric halts melatonin production and it also contains important antioxidant and antibacterial properties so that it is helpful to the overall health of the skin. Turmeric is a natural sunscreen and that is found in many manufactured beauty products (From: ehow.com)

Porocedure:

1-Mix equal parts of turmeric powder and cucumber juice until it makes a smooth paste or cream. If the cream is too dry or too wet to easily apply to the skin, then add a bit more juice or turmeric powder

2- Apply the turmeric cream to the body. Leave it on for approximately 15 minutes. You can add Nano Solution to make a Nano Cream.

Washing in turmeric improves skin complexion and also reduces hair growth on body. Nowadays there are lots of herbal products in the market in which main herb used is turmeric as natural ingredient. These constitute home remedies for skin and hair problems.

Natural cleansers like milk with turmeric powder are effective natural cosmetics in themselves; it brings a healthy glow to the skin and makes them beautiful. They also help to restore or maintain youth by controlling wrinkle and crease formation on the surface of the skin. **Turmeric can also benefit skin conditions including: eczema, psoriasis and acne.**

Phytochemical Compounds Inside Turmeric & Their Effects on Health

Chemical Compounds and their Activities in Turmeric

Here is a list of the most important chemical compounds found in turmeric together with their benefit effects on different health issues (from Duke's Phytochemical Database:

In his book Dr. Dukes Essential Herbs, Dr. James Duke discusses "turmeric's medicinal power" emphasizing certain constituents including the following:

- **Antioxidants** including vitamins C and E, several carotenoids, curcumin, and related compounds called curcuminoids.
- **Cyclooxygenase-2 (COX 2) inhibitors**, effective at blocking inflammation, especially inflammation caused by arthritis and gout.
- **Curcumin** is one of the above mentioned antioxidants. It neutralizes some cancer causing substances and acts as an anti-mutagenic stopping very early changes in cells that can turn to cancer. Curcumin also protects the heart, is antiviral (and thus may be useful to HIV patients), and is a cell growth generator speeding up the healing of wounds.
- **Cineole** which stimulates the central nervous system, is antiseptic, is expectorant, and eliminates gas.

. *There are a total of 92 constituents in this list and most of them have known activities, which overlap with the activities of other constituents.*
Dr. Duke's Phytochemical and Ethnobotanical Databases
Chemicals and their Biological Activities in: Curcuma longa L. (Zingiberaceae) – Indian Saffron, Turmeric:

1, 8-CINEOLE Rhizome 30 - 720 ppm
Allelopathic; Allergenic; Anesthetic; Anthelminthic; Antiacetylcholinesterase; Antiallergic; Antibacterial; Antibronchitic;Anticatarrh; Anticholinesterase; Antifatigue; Antihalitosic; Antilaryngitic; Antipharyngitic; Antirhinitic; Antiseptic; Antispasmodic; Antistaphylococcic;Antitussive; Candidicide; Choleretic; CNS-Stimulant; Convulsant; Counterirritant; Cytochrome-P450-Inducer; Degranulant; Dentifrice;Edemagenic inj; Expectorant; FLavor; Fungicide; Gram(+)icide; Gram(-)icide; Hepatotonic; Herbicide; Hypotensive;Inflammatory inj; Insectifuge; Irritant; Myorelaxant; Nematicide; Neurotoxic; P450-Inducer; Perfume; Pesticide; Rubefacient; Secretogogue; Sedative;
Spasmogenic; Surfactant; Testosterone-Hydroxylase-Inducer; Trichomonicide

2-HYDROXY-METHYL-ANTHRAQUINONE Rhizome:
Antileukemic; Cytotoxic

4-HYDROXY-CINNAMOYL-(FERULOYL)-METHANE Rhizome 180 ppm;
No activity reported.

ALPHA-PINENE Essential Oil 5, 300 ppm;

THE 50 MIRACLE CURES OF CURCUMIN

Allelochemic; Allergenic; Antibacterial; Antifeedant; Antiflu; Antiinflammatory; Antiviral; Cancer-Preventive; Coleoptophile; Expectorant; Flavor; Herbicide; Insectifuge ; Insectiphile; Irritant; Perfumery; Pesticide; Sedative; Spasmogenic; Tranquilizer

ALPHA-TERPINEOL Rhizome:
ACE-Inhibitor 100 ug/ml (weak activity); Aldose-Reductase-Inhibitor; Antibacterial; Anticariogenic; Antiseptic;FLavor; Motor-Depressant; Nematicide; Perfumery; Pesticide; Sedative; Termiticide

AR-TURMERONE Rhizome 5, 800 ppm;
Antihemorrhagic; Antiinflammatory; Antilymphocytic; Antiophidic; Antitumor; Insectifuge; Pesticide

ARABINOSE Rhizome 10, 000 ppm;
No activity reported.

ASCORBIC-ACID Rhizome 293 ppm;
Acidulant; Aldose-Reductase-Inhibitor; Analgesic; Antiaggregant; Antiaging; Antiarthritic ; Antiasthmatic; Antiatherosclerotic; Antibacterial; Anticataract; Anticold; AntiCrohn's; Antidecubitic; Antidepressant; Antidiabetic; Antidote (Aluminum); Antidote (Cadmium);Antidote (Lead); Antidote (Paraquat); Antieczemic; Antiedemic 1 g/man/day; Antiencephalitic; Antigingivitic; Antiglaucomic;Antihemorrhagic; Antihepatitic; Antihepatotoxic; Antiherpetic; Antihistaminic; Antiinfertility ; Antiinflammatory; Antilepric 1.5 g/man/day; Antimeasles; Antimigraine; Antimutagenic; Antinitrosic 1 g/man/day; Antiobesity;Antiorchitic; Antiosteoarthritic; Antiosteoporotic; Antioxidant; Antiparkinsonian; Antiparotitic;Antiperiodontitic; Antipneumonic; Antipodriac; Antipoliomyelitic; Antipyretic; Antiradicular; Antiscorbutic; Antiseptic ; Antishingles; Antisyndrome-X; Antitumor (Lung); Antiulcer; Antiviral; Apoptotic;Asthma-preventive; Beta-Glucuronidase-Inhibitor; Cancer-Preventive; Cold-preventive; Collagenic;Detoxicant; Diuretic; Fistula-Preventive; Hypocholesterolemic; Hypoglycemic; Hypotensive;immunostimulant; Interferonogenic; Lithogenic; Mucolytic; Pesticide; Uricosuric; Urinary-Acidulant; Vulnerary

ASH Rhizome 9, 000 - 148, 000 ppm
No activity reported.

AZULENE Rhizome:
Antiallergic; Antibacterial 500 ppm; Antihistaminic; Antiinflammatory; Antipyretic; Antiseptic; Antispasmodic; Antiulcer ;Hepatoregenerative; Pesticide

BETA-CAROTENE Rhizome:
Allergenic; Androgenic?; Antiacne; Antiaging; Antiasthmatic; Anticarcinomic; Anticoronary; Antihyperkeratotic; Antiichythyotic; Antileukoplakic; Antilupus; Antimastitic; Antimutagenic; Antioxidant; Antiozenic; Antiphotophobic;Antipityriasic; AntiPMS; Antiporphyric; Antipsoriac; Antiradicular; Antistress; Antitumor; Antiulcer; Antixerophthalmic; Cancer-Preventive; Colorant; Immunostimulant; Interferon-Synergist; Mucogenic; Phagocytotic;Prooxidant; Thymoprotective; Ubiquiot

BETA-PINENE Essential Oil 2, 700 ppm;
Allergenic; Antiinflammatory; Antiseptic; Candidicide; FLavor; Herbicide; Insectifuge; Perfumery; Pesticide; Spasmogenic

BETA-SESQUIPHELLANDRENE Rhizome:
Antirhinoviral; Antiulcer; Expectorant; Pesticide

BIS-DESMETHOXYCURCUMIN Rhizome 67 - 27, 000 ppm
Antiangiogenic; Anticholeretic; Antiinflammatory

BORNEOL Rhizome:

Allelochemic; Analgesic; Antiacetylcholine; Antibronchitic; Antifeedant; Antiinflammatory; Antipyretic; Antispasmodic, CNS-Stimulant; CNS-Toxic; FLavor; Hepatoprotective; Herbicide; Inhalant; Insect-Repellent; Insectifuge; Irritant; Myorelaxant; Nematicide; Perfumery; Pesticide; Sedative

BORON Root 1 - 6 ppm
Androgenic; Antiosteoarthritic; Antiosteoporotic; Estrogenic

CAFFEIC-ACID Rhizome 5 ppm;
Aldose-Reductase-Inhibitor); Allergenic; Analgesic; Antiadenoviral; Antiaggregant; Antibacterial; Anticancer; Anticarcinogenic; Antiedemic; Antiflu; Antigonadotropic; Antihemolytic; Antihepatoadenomic; Antihepatotoxic; Antiherpetic; Antihistaminic; AntiHIV; Antihypercholesterolemic; Antiinflammatory; Antileukotriene; Antimutagenic; Antinitrosaminic; Antiophidic; Antioxidant quercetin ; Antiperoxidant; Antiprostaglandin; Antiradicular ;quercetin; Antiseptic; Antispasmodic; Antistomatitic; Antisunburn; Antithiamin; Antithyroid; Antitumor; Antitumor-Promoter; Antiulcerogenic; Antivaccinia; Antiviral; Calcium-Antagonist; Cancer-Preventive; Cholagogue; Choleretic; Clastogenic; CNS-Active; Cocarcinogenic; Collagen-Sparing; Cytoprotective; Cytotoxic; Diuretic; DNA-Active; Fungicide; Hepatocarcinogenic (in the absence of alcohol); Hepatoprotective; Hepatotropic; Immunostimulant; Insectifuge; Lipoxygenase-Inhibitor Lyase-Inhibitor ; Metal-Chelator; Ornithine-Decarboxylase-Inhibitor; Pesticide; Prooxidant; Prostaglandigenic; Sedative; Sunscreen; Tumorigenic; Vulnerary; Xanthine-Oxidase-Inhibitor

CALCIUM Rhizome 270 - 2, 898 ppm
Antiallergic; Antianxiety; Antiatherosclerotic; Antidepressant; Antidote (Aluminum); Antidote (Lead); Antihyperkinetic; Antiinsomniac; Antiosteoporotic; Antiperiodontitic; AntiPMS; Antitic; Hypocholesterolemic; Hypotensive

CAPRYLIC-ACID Rhizome:
Candidicide; Fungicide; Irritant; Pesticide

CARBOHYDRATES Rhizome 79, 000 - 829, 000 ppm
No activity reported.

CARYOPHYLLENE Essential Oil:
Aldose-Reductase-Inhibitor; Antiacne; Antiasthmatic; Antibacterial; Anticariogenic; Antiedemic; Antifeedant; Antiinflammatory; Antispasmodic; Antistreptococcic; Antitumor; FLavor; Insectifuge; Perfumery; Pesticide; Termitifuge

CHROMIUM Rhizome 6 ppm;
AntiAGE; Antiaging; Antiatherosclerotic; Anticorneotic; Antidiabetic; Antidote (Lead); Antiglycosuric; Antiobesity; Antisyndrome-X; Antitriglyceride; Hypocholesterolemic ; Hypoglycemic; Hypotensive; Insulinogenic

CINEOLE Essential Oil 29, 200 ppm;
No activity reported.

CINNAMIC-ACID Rhizome:
Aldose-Reductase-Inhibitor Allergenic; Anesthetic; Antibacterial; Antiinflammatory; Antimutagenic; Antispasmodic; Cancer-Preventive; Choleretic; Dermatitigenic; FLavor; Fungicide; Herbicide; Laxative; Lipoxygenase-Inhibitor; Pesticide; Vermifuge

COBALT Rhizome 1 ppm;
Cardiomyopathogenic; Erythrocytogenic

COPPER Rhizome 6 - 17 ppm

THE 50 MIRACLE CURES OF CURCUMIN — 155

Antiarthritic; Antidiabetic; Antiinflammatory; Antinociceptive; Contraceptive; Hypocholesterolemic; Schizophrenigenic

CURCUMENE Essential Oil 121, 700 ppm;
No activity reported.

CURCUMENOL Essential Oil 21, 300 ppm;
Anticancer; Emetic

CURCUMIN Rhizome 9 - 38, 888 ppm
12-Lipoxygenase-Inhibitor; 5-Lipoxygenase-Inhibitor; Antiadenomacarcinogenic -; Antiaflatoxin; Antiaggregant; Antiangiogenic; Antiarachidonate; Antiarthritic; Antiasthmatic; Antiatherosclerotic; Antibacterial; Antibronchitic; Anticancer (Breast); Anticancer (Colon); Anticancer (Duodenum); Anticancer (Mammary); Anticancer (Skin); Anticataract; Anticholecystosic;Anticolitic; AntiCrohn's; AntiEBV; Antieczemic; Antiedemic Antihepatotic; AntiHIV; Antiinflammatory ; Antiintegrase; Antiischemic; Antileukemic; Antileukotriene; Antilithic; Antilymphomic;Antimelanomic; Antimetastatic; Antimutagenic; Antinitrosaminic; Antioxidant; Antiprostaglandin; Antipsoriatic; Antispasmodic; Antithrombotic; Antithromboxane; Antitumor (Colon); Antitumor-Promoter;Antiulcer; Antiviral; Apoptotic; Cancer-Preventive; Cardiodepressant; Chelator;Cholagogue; Choleretic; COX-2-Inhibitor /; Cyclooxygenase-Inhibitor; Cytochrome-P450-Inhibitor; Cytotoxic;
Deodorant; Detoxicant; Dye; Fibrinolytic; Fungicide; Hepatoprotective; Hypocholesterolemic Hypolipidemic; Hypotensive; Immunostimulant; Litholytic; Metal-Chelator; Ornithine-Decarboxylase-Inhibitor;Pesticide; Phototoxic; Prostaglandin-Synthesis-Inhibitor; Protease-Inhibitor; Protein-Kinase-Inhibitor; Pulmonoprotective; Quinone-Reductase-Inducer; Ulcerogenic .

CURDIONE Essential Oil 11, 900 ppm;
Anticancer (Cervix); Antileukopenic; Antisarcomic; Antitumor; AntiX-Radiation

DESMETHOXYCURCUMIN Rhizome 500 - 11, 100 ppm
No activity reported.

DI-P-COUMAROYL-METHANE Rhizome:
Cytotoxic; Hepatoprotective

DICINNAMOYLMETHANE Rhizome:
Choleretic

DIFERULOYL-METHANE Rhizome:
Cytotoxic

EO Rhizome 3, 000 - 72, 000 ppm
No activity reported.

EUGENOL Essential Oil 2, 100 ppm;
Allergenic; Analgesic; Anesthetic; Antiaggregant; Antiarachidonate; Antibacterial; Anticonvulsant; Antiedemic 100;Antifeedant; Antiinflammatory; Antimitotic; Antimutagenic; Antinitrosating; Antioxidant; Antiprostaglandin ; Antipyretic 3 ml/man/day; Antiradicular; Antiseptic 3 ml/man/day; Antispasmodic; Antithromboxane; Antitumor; Antiulcer;
Apifuge; Calcium-Antagonist; Cancer-Preventive; Candidicide; Carminative; Choleretic; CNS-Depressant; Cytochrome-P450-Inhibitor; Cytotoxic; Dermatitigenic; Enterorelaxant; FLavor; Fungicide;Hepatoprotective; Herbicide; Insecticide; Insectifuge; Irritant; Juvabional; Larvicide; Motor-Depressant; Nematicide; Neurotoxic; Perfumery; Pesticide; Prostaglandin-Synthesis-Inhibitor; Sedative; Trichomonicide; Trichomonistat; Trypsin-Enhancer; Ulcerogenic; Vermifuge

FAT Rhizome 18, 000 - 153, 000 ppm
No activity reported.

FERULOYL-P-COUMAROYL-METHANE Rhizome: Cytotoxic

FIBER Rhizome 9, 000 - 84, 000 ppm
Antidiabetic; Antiobesity; Antitumor; Antiulcer; Cancer-Preventive; Cardioprotective; Hypocholesterolemic; Hypotensive; Laxative

FRUCTOSE Rhizome 120, 000 ppm;
Antialcoholic; Antidiabetic; Antihangover; Antiketotic; Antinauseant; Laxative; Neoplastic; Sweetener 2 x glucose

GLUCOSE Rhizome 280, 000 ppm;
Acetylcholinergic; Antiedemic; Antihepatotoxic; Antiketotic; Antivaricose; Hyperglycemic; Memory-Enhancer

GUAIACOL Rhizome:
Anesthetic; Antibacterial; Antidermatitic; Antieczemic; Antiesophagitic; Antiseptic; Antituberculic; Cardiotonic; Expectorant;; Insectifuge; Pesticide; Prostaglandin-Synthesis-Inhibitor

IRON Rhizome 121 - 467 ppm
Antiakathisic; Antianemic; Anticheilitic; Antimenorrhagic

ISOBORNEOL Rhizome Essent. Oil 200 ppm;
Insectifuge; Motor-Stimulant; Nematicide; Pesticide; Sedative

L-ALPHA-CURCUMENE Rhizome 18, 000 ppm;
No activity reported.

L-BETA-CURCUMENE Rhizome 18, 000 ppm;
No activity reported.

LIMONENE Essential Oil 2, 300 ppm;
AChE-Inhibitor; Allelochemic; Allergenic; Antiacetylcholinesterase; Antialzheimeran; Antibacterial; Anticancer; Antifeedant; Antiflu; Antilithic; Antimutagenic; Antiseptic; Antispasmodic ; Antitumor; Antitumor (Breast); Antitumor (Pancreas); Antitumor (Prostate); Antiviral; Cancer-Preventive; Candidistat; Chemopreventive; Enterocontractant; Expectorant; FLavor; Fungiphilic; Fungistat; Herbicide; Insecticide; Insectifuge; Irritant; Nematicide IC=100 ug/ml; Ornithine-Decarboxylase-Inhibitor Pesticide; Photosensitizer; Sedative

LINALOL Essential Oil 1, 600 ppm;
Anti-diabetic.

MANGANESE Rhizome 33 - 78 ppm
Antialcoholic; Antianemic; Antidiabetic; Antidiscotic; Antidyskinetic; Antiepileptic; Antiototic; Antisyndrome-X; Hypoglycemic

NIACIN Rhizome 5 - 62 ppm
Allergenic; Antiacrodynic; Antiallergic; Antiamblyopic; Antianginal; Antichilblain; Anticonvulsant; Antidermatitic; Antidysphagic;Antiepileptic; Antihistaminic; Antihyperactivity; Antiinsomnic; AntiMeniere's; Antineuralgic; Antiparkinsonian   ; Antipellagric; Antiscotomic; Antispasmodic; Antivertigo; Cancer-Preventive; Hepatoprotective; Hypoglycemic; Hypolipidemic; Sedative; Serotoninergic; Vasodilator

THE 50 MIRACLE CURES OF CURCUMIN

NICKEL Rhizome 3.8 ppm;
Antiadrenalinic; Anticirrhotic?; Insulin-Sparing

O-COUMARIC-ACID Leaf:
Antibacterial; Fungicide; Pesticide

P-COUMARIC-ACID Rhizome 345 ppm;
Aldose-Reductase-Inhibitor Allelopathic; Antibacterial; Antifertility; Antihepatotoxic; Antioxidant;Antiperoxidant; Antispasmodic; Antitumor; Cancer-Preventive; Choleretic; Cytotoxic; Diaphoretic?; Fungicide; Lipoxygenase-Inhibitor; Pesticide; Prostaglandigenic; Prostaglandin-Synthesis-Inhibitor

P-CYMENE Rhizome:
Analgesic; Antiacetylcholinesterase; Antibacterial; Antiflu; Antirheumatalgic; Antiviral; FLavor; Fungicide; Herbicide; Insectifuge; Pesticide; Trichomonicide

P-METHOXY-CINNAMIC-ACID Rhizome 360 ppm;
Antipyretic; Fungicide; Hemolytic; Hypoglycemic; Pesticide

P-TOLYMETHYLCARBINOL Rhizome 500 - 1, 750 ppm
Cholagogue

PHOSPHORUS Rhizome 640 - 6, 307 ppm
Antiosteoporotic; Immunostimulant; Osteogenic

POTASSIUM Rhizome 4, 870 - 41, 271 ppm
Antiarrhythmic; Antidepressant; Antifatigue; Antihypertensive; Antispasmodic; Cardiotoxic

PROTEIN Rhizome 12, 000 - 306, 000 ppm
No activity reported.

PROTOCATECHUIC-ACID Leaf:
Antiarrhythmic; Antiasthmatic; Antibacterial; Antihepatotoxic; Antiherpetic; Antiinflammatory; Antiischemic; Antiophidic; Antioxidant; Antiperoxidant; Antiradicular; Antispasmodic; Antitussive; Antiviral; Fungicide; Immunostimulant; Pesticide; Phagocytotic; Prostaglandigenic; Secretogogue; Ubiquiot

RIBOFLAVIN Rhizome 12 ppm;
Antiarabiflavinotic ; Anticarpal-Tunnel; Anticataract; Anticheilitic; Antidecubitic; Antiglossitic; Antikeratitic; Antimigraine; Antipellagric; Antiphotophobic; Cancer-Preventive

SODIUM Rhizome 30 - 4, 290 ppm
Hypertensive

SYRINGIC-ACID Leaf:
Antioxidant; Ubiquiot

TERPINENE Essential Oil 27, 200 ppm;
No activity reported.

TERPINEOL Essential Oil 500 ppm;
Antiallergenic; Antiasthmatic; Antibacterial; Antiseptic; Antitussive; Cholagogue; Expectorant; Insectifuge; Perfumery; Pesticide

THIAMIN Rhizome 8 ppm;
Analgesic; Antialcoholic; Antialzheimeran; Antianorectic; Antibackache; Antiberiberi; Anticardiospasmic; Anticolitic; Antidecubitic; Antideliriant; Antiencephalopathic; Antifatigue; Antigastritic; Antiheartburn; Antiherpetic; Antimigraine; Antimyocarditic; Antineuralgic; Antineurasthenic; Antineuritic; Antineuropathic; Antipoliomyelitic; Insectifuge; Pesticide

TURMERONE Rhizome 1, 800 - 43, 200 ppm
Choleretic; Hepatotonic; Insectifuge; Pesticide

UKONAN-A Rhizome 33 - 6, 600 ppm
Immunostimulant; Phagocytotic; RES-Activator

VANILLIC-ACID Leaf:
Aldose-Reductase-Inhibitor; Anthelminthic; Antibacterial; Anticancer; Antifatigue; Antiinflammatory; Antioxidant; Antiradicular 7 x quercetin; Antisickling; Antitumor; Antitumor-Promoter; Ascaricide; Cancer-Preventive; Choleretic; Immunosuppressant; Laxative; Pesticide; Ubiquiot

WATER Rhizome 133, 000 ppm;
No activity reported.

ZINC Rhizome 22 ppm;
Antiacne; Antiacrodermatitic; Antialopecic; Antialzheimeran; Antianorexic; Antiarthritic ; Anticanker; Anticataract; Anticoeliac; Anticold; Anticolitic; Anticoronary; AntiCrohn's; Antidandruff; Antidiabetic; Antidote (Cadmium); Antieczemic; Antiencephalopathic; Antiepileptic; Antifuruncular; Antiherpetic; Antiimpotence; Antiinfective; Antiinfertility ; Antiinsomniac; Antilepric; Antileukonychic; Antiobesity; Antiplaque; Antiprolactin; Antiprostatitic; Antirheumatic; Antispare-Tire ; Antistomatitic; Antisyndrome-X; Antitinnitic; Antitriglyceride; Antiulcer days; Antiviral; Astringent; Copper-Antagonist; Deodorant; Hypotensive; Immunostimulant; Immunosuppressant; Insulinogenic; Leptingenic; Mucogenic; Pesticide; Spermigenic; Testosteronigenic; Trichomonicide; Vulnerary

ZINGIBERENE Rhizome 750 - 18, 000 ppm
Antirhinoviral; Antiulcer; Carminative; Insecticide; Perfumery; Pesticide

ppm = parts per million

It is very clear from the list of chemical compounds present in coriander and their action that coriander inner composition offers us huge number of health benefits for:

Diabetes, Cholesterol, Triglycerides, Gout, Kidney, Liver, Heart, Ulcer, Gallbladder, Prostate, Joints, Cancer, High Blood Pressure, Weight Loss, Asthma……etc.
Chapters of the book show us in details about these health benefits.

About the Author
Awad Mansour, Ph.D.

Professor of Chemical Engineering & Pharmaceutical Industry
profmansour@gmail.com   www.pharmatech1.com
www.magicperfume.net
www.yarmouktoqrcure.com   www.profmansour.com
www.swineflu-cures.com

PERSONAL : D.O.B : March, 13, 1951
EDUCATION : B.Sc. in Chemical Engineering, Baghdad University 1975, M.Sc. & Ph.D. in Chemical Engineering, University of Tulsa, Oklahoma,U.S.A., 1980.
TEACHING EXPERIENCE: 1980-2008 with Yarmouk ,Jordan University of Science & Technology.
1993-1994 : University of Akron,Ohio,U.S.A. Chairman of of Chemical Engineering & Pharmaceutical
   Department at Jordan University of Science & Technology 1989-1990.

PUBLICATIONS: *100 PUBLISHED PAPERS IN REFEREED JOURNALS*
PATENTS IN POLYMER, WATER & OIL INDUSTRY:
A Carry-Along Toilet "CARRYLET" a joint author with A.B. Shahalam M.O., Othman **registered in JORDAN, No. 87-1307, 1987.,**Multi-Purpose Surfactant/Detergent for Oil Recovery from Water, Oil Spills, Tar Sands, Beach Sand and Shale Oil, Drag Reduction and Emulsification Processes, Kansas, (GemTech Solvents 1983-93),
A New Drag Reducing Additive for Crude Oil Pipelines & Sanitary Sewers, Certified by the University of Akron, Ohio, U.S.A 1983-1995,A New Heat Reducing Additive for District Heating, HV AC Systems and Hydro-Power Plants, High Tech Technology, Cleveland & University of Akron, Akron, Ohio, U.S.A. 1993-1995.
A New Cold Technology for Shale Oil Extraction at Room Temperature,2006,
A New Surfactant to Separate Oil from Canadian Oil Sand at Room Temperature,. Edmonton, Alberta, Canada, 2006,New Surfactants to Solve Oil Spill Problems on Beaches and in the Sea, Certified by Alberta Research,Edmonton, Canada ,2001.
New Polymer Composites, Case Western & Reserve University, Cleveland, Ohio, U.S.A. (1993-1994).A NEW Cold Biodiesel Production Using A New Efficient Technolgy; JORDA, 2008,New Nano Water Elecrolysis to Produce Commercial Hydrogen; Jordan,2008,New Ultrasonic Water Elecrolysis to Produce Commercial

Hydrogen; Jordan,2008,New Nano Double Strength Concrete; JORDAN, 2009,A New Efficient Motor Oil Additive, JORDAN,2008.

PATENTS IN HERBAL MEDICINE
PRESS TECH: For Hypertension,AZMA TECH for Asthma.DIA TECH 2000: for Diabetes I & II. RENO TECH 2000: The First Cure for Kidney Failure. MG10,MG20 : for Cancer. IMU TECH&IMUFAST : for HIV, Hepatitis C & B. SPLEENO TECH for Spleen,VIA TECH: for Sex,PSORIA. TECH, LIV TECH, CHOLES TECH , PROSTA TECH,MC10 for malaria,JOINT TECH,RELAX U

CHEM. ENG. & COMPUTER BOOKS: DRAG & HEAT REDUCTION, HTT, Ohio. U.S.A. 1995,AMAZON.COM
Chemical Separation,ed. J.C..King,U.S.A.,Chapter on Adsorption.217-237(1986)
60 COMPUTER BOOKS: Published 1983-2008

HEALTH & MEDICINAL BOOKS:
DO NOT BE AFRAID OF SWINE FLU,AMAZON.COM,2009
The 50 Miracle Cures of Coriander, AMAZON.COM,2009
The 50 Miracle Cures of Curcumin, Health Tech Book Series,2009
60 HEALTH BOOKS ARE COMING IN U.S.A.

MEMBERSHIP IN SCIENTIFIC AND PROFESSIONAL SOCIETIES

- American Institute of Chemical Engineers and Jordanian Engineers' Society.
- AMERICAN HERB RESEARCH FOUNDATION
- AMERICAN HEALTH SCIENCES INSTITUTE
- INTERNATIONAL SOCIETY OH PHARMACEUTICAL ENGINEERING
- NEW YORK ACADEMY OF SCIENCES